Nuclear Medicine Manual on Gynaecological Cancers and Other Female Malignancies

Angela Collarino
Sergi Vidal-Sicart
Renato A. Valdés Olmos
Editors

Nuclear Medicine Manual on Gynaecological Cancers and Other Female Malignancies

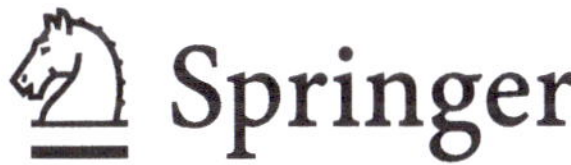

Editors
Angela Collarino
Nuclear Medicine Unit
Fondazione Policlinico
Universitario A. Gemelli IRCCS
Rome, Italy

Sergi Vidal-Sicart
Nuclear Medicine
Hospital Clinic of Barcelona
Catalonia, Barcelona, Spain

Renato A. Valdés Olmos
Radiology
Leiden University Medical Center
Leiden, The Netherlands

ISBN 978-3-031-05499-0 ISBN 978-3-031-05497-6 (eBook)
https://doi.org/10.1007/978-3-031-05497-6

This Springer imprint is published by the registered company Springer Nature Switzerland AG
The registered company address is: Gewerbestrasse 11, 6330 Cham, Switzerland

Foreword

Cancer is a prominent cause of mortality in both economically developed and underdeveloped countries and the number of patients seeking care for these malignancies is increasing. Unfortunately, the burden is expected to grow globally due to increasing age of the population. Breast cancer is the most common malignancy in women, and other female malignancies such as endometrial cancer, ovarian cancer and cervical cancer are among the top 10 most common cancers in women worldwide. Therefore, this book is primarily notable for its focus on a very important public health problem.

The rising incidence of cancer worldwide has prompted many improvements to current care. Nuclear medicine procedures have been major contributors in the diagnosis at different stages of the disease, such as early lesion detection, staging, monitoring and predicting response to therapy, as well as detecting progression, recurrence or metastases. Developments in instrumentation and the introduction of new radiopharmaceuticals have offered new possibilities that have helped to improve the different diagnostic aspects. Another notable feature of this book is that it analyses in detail the clinical utility of different nuclear medicine techniques in each of the malignancies. Among them we should highlight the sentinel node procedure, which includes radiotracer administration, preoperative lymphoscintigraphy and intraoperative detection, as well as some specific modalities (ROLL, RSL …). In addition, the utility of other diagnostic imaging modalities such as SPECT/CT, PET/CT or PEM is well described, focusing again on their clinical usefulness.

So here we have a book which offers clear intentions of clinical application. Described as a handbook, this is even more impactful as it implies that this is a book which one should always have in hand. The way it has been structured by chapters, according to the different tumours, seems to me to be very effective. Each chapter begins with a description of general aspects relating to that specific tumour (anatomy, types and subtypes, lymphatic drainage, TNM classification, etc.) followed by the different nuclear medicine techniques which could be useful in each case.

The multidisciplinary vision of the book makes it interesting to both specialists in nuclear medicine, radiology or gynaecology. In my opinion, it can also be useful for future specialists, i.e. residents in training, because of its global vision of the tumours it describes and also for its detailed description of the diagnostic techniques.

The authors are recognized leaders in this field. I have had the opportunity to work with some of them, and I want to acknowledge that they are great professionals and great people. We should recognize the effort made, as a team, which demonstrates both their knowledge and experience.

In summary, the book deals with an important public health problem in women and has clear intentions of clinical application. Its format is both practical and manageable, and its authors are leaders on the subject. It is a book which responds to the need to update knowledge and to disseminate any important future developments in a concise and enjoyable way. We could not want for more.

Hospital Clínic
University of Barcelona,
Barcelona, Spain

Francesca Pons

Preface

Although female-related malignancies such as breast cancer and gynaecological neoplasms constitute an important part of clinical oncology, there are no nuclear medicine books specifically oriented to this topic. The book *Nuclear Medicine Manual on Gynaecological Cancers and Other Female Malignancies* has been designed to build a bridge between female cancer oncology and nuclear medicine in order to fill this hiatus.

In the last 30 years, multidisciplinary procedures have gradually gained in popularity in clinical oncology. One of these procedures is sentinel node biopsy which has become standard of care for staging in various malignancies. In female-related cancer, due to its limited morbidity and high accuracy, the sentinel node procedure has replaced axillary lymph node dissection in staging the axilla in patients with early breast cancer and no evidence of regional lymph node metastases. A similar trajectory can be observed for gynaecological cancers which started in the nineties of the past century with the validation of the procedure in vulvar cancer, followed in this century by its extension to cervical and endometrial cancer. In these latter malignancies, the incorporation of SPECT/CT has played an important role by providing helpful information to localize sentinel nodes in relation to blood vessels, muscles and other anatomical structures.

Apart from the sentinel node procedure, PET/CT with ^{18}F-FDG emerged as another modality with increasing clinical applications. Particularly for breast cancer and gynaecological malignancies ^{18}F-FDG PET/CT has demonstrated high diagnostic accuracy for the evaluation of regional and distant metastases principally in patients with locally advanced cancer. In many cases, the use of this modality may change clinical management from curative to palliative. Compared with sentinel node biopsy ^{18}F-FDG PET/CT has poorer sensitivity for regional nodal metastases, but it contributes significantly to clinical staging by demonstrating occult distant nodal involvement as well as pleural, hepatic, splenic, adrenal and pelvic metastases. On the other hand, the high positive predictive value of the modality leads to a better risk stratification by estimating tumour load which, for instance, may be of application in the axilla for breast cancer and in the pelvis for gynaecological cancer. This may be helpful to determine which patients need additional radiotherapy.

The success of sentinel node biopsy and ^{18}F-FDG PET/CT has led to their incorporation in guidelines and recommendations of diverse national and international scientific societies. It has also facilitated the development of other interventional nuclear medicine tools concerning both radioguided surgery with specific devices and hybrid tomographic imaging with different PET tracers. The role of these new techniques is pointed out in the corresponding chapters of this manual.

The structure of this edition is organized as a handbook. It aims to enable readers to have quick access to interventional nuclear medicine applications in the field of female malignancies. The book is divided into five chapters. Every chapter includes numerous panels with specific topics richly illustrated with schematic images and teaching cases. Chapter 1 firstly summarizes data on worldwide statistics, types and subtypes as well as TNM staging of breast cancer to subsequently discuss aspects like lymphatic drainage, radiotracer administration, preoperative sentinel node mapping and intraoperative detection. The chapter also includes specific panels on radioguided occult lesion localization (ROLL), radioguided seed localization (RSL) and targeted lymph node biopsy. Last, the chapter discusses not only the role of ^{18}F-FDG and other PET tracers using both PET/CT and dedicated devices in breast cancer but also the contribution of molecular breast imaging with ^{99m}Tc-sestamibi and the feasibility of new integrated interventional nuclear medicine-based strategies for axillary management. Chapter 2 concerns vulvar cancer with extended information about the methodological aspects of sentinel node biopsy and its clinical indication. These topics are preceded by an overview of lymphatic drainage, tumour types, FIGO classification and utility of SPECT/CT. The chapter also discusses the role of ^{18}F-FDG PET/CT and finally includes the contribution of nuclear medicine to the management of vaginal cancer. Chapter 3 introduces cervical cancer by presenting general aspects like anatomy, lymphatic drainage, tumour types and FIGO classification. Subsequently, the chapter summarizes methodological and conceptual aspects of lymphatic mapping and sentinel node imaging emphasizing the synergistic role of lymphoscintigraphy and SPECT/CT. Finally, the chapter discusses the utility of ^{18}F-FDG PET/CT for detection of regional and distant metastases. Different from malignancies affecting vulva and cervix, where tracer administration has been well-standardized in endometrial cancer controversies concerning tracer administration remain. The different routes for tracer injection are discussed in Chap. 4, following the presentation of other items like lymphatic drainage, tumour types, TNM classification, gamma camera imaging including lymphoscintigraphy and SPECT/CT and the use of ROLL and RSL. Particular attention is given to the role of ^{18}F-FDG PET/CT in clinical staging. Chapter 5, the last chapter of the book, concerns ovarian cancer, which is the most recent clinical application of both sentinel node biopsy and ^{18}F-FDG PET/CT.

The content of all chapters has been prepared by international experts in radioguided surgery, lymphatic mapping and hybrid tomographic imaging incorporating state-of-the-art information concerning clinical indications and technological advances. The editors have preferred to compose the materials following a handbook model rather than a textbook one. Together with a book structure based on specific topics summarizing information and data, every chapter incorporates special designed illustrations and selected key references per panel. The numbers of the references appear in parentheses at the end of every panel, and the references are fully cited as suggested readings at the end of every chapter.

Originally conceived during the congress of the European Association of Nuclear Medicine held in Barcelona in 2019, this first version of the book not only represents the cooperative efforts of editors and authors, but also the confluence of various generations of specialists in nuclear medicine and clinical oncology. The editors hope to continue this cooperation in future editions of the book.

The editors also thank the support of Springer for making it possible to publish this manual supporting its specific technical levels and concept.

Rome, Italy — Angela Collarino
Barcelona, Spain — Sergi Vidal-Sicart
Leiden, The Netherlands — Renato A. Valdés Olmos
January 2022

Contents

1 Breast Cancer

Renato A. Valdés Olmos,
Lenka M. Pereira Arias-Bouda,
Daphne D. D. Rietbergen, and
Jos A. van der Hage

1.1 Breast Cancer Statistics

According to the estimates of cancer incidence and mortality produced by the International Agency for Research and Cancer for 2020, female breast cancer has surpassed lung cancer as the most commonly diagnosed cancer with an estimated 2.3 million new cases (11.7% of all cancer cases). Breast cancer is the most commonly diagnosed female cancer in 159 countries and is the leading cause of cancer death in 110 countries. With 685,000 deaths breast cancer is, worldwide, the fifth leading cause of cancer mortality. Incidence rates are 88% higher in transitioned countries than in transitioning countries (55.9 and 29.7 per 100,000, respectively) with Belgium as the country with the world's highest incidence. However, women living in transitioning countries have 17% higher mortality rates compared with women in transitioned countries (15.0 and 12.8 per 100,000, respectively) with Barbados as the country with the highest mortality in the world.

R. A. Valdés Olmos (✉)
Radiology, Leiden University Medical Center, Leiden, The Netherlands
e-mail: R.A.Valdes_Olmos@lumc.nl

L. M. Pereira Arias-Bouda · D. D. D. Rietbergen
J. A. van der Hage
Department of Radiology, Section of Nuclear Medicine and Interventional Molecular Imaging Laboratory, Leiden University Medical Centre, Leiden, The Netherlands

A. Collarino et al. (eds.), *Nuclear Medicine Manual on Gynaecological Cancers and Other Female Malignancies*, https://doi.org/10.1007/978-3-031-05497-6_1

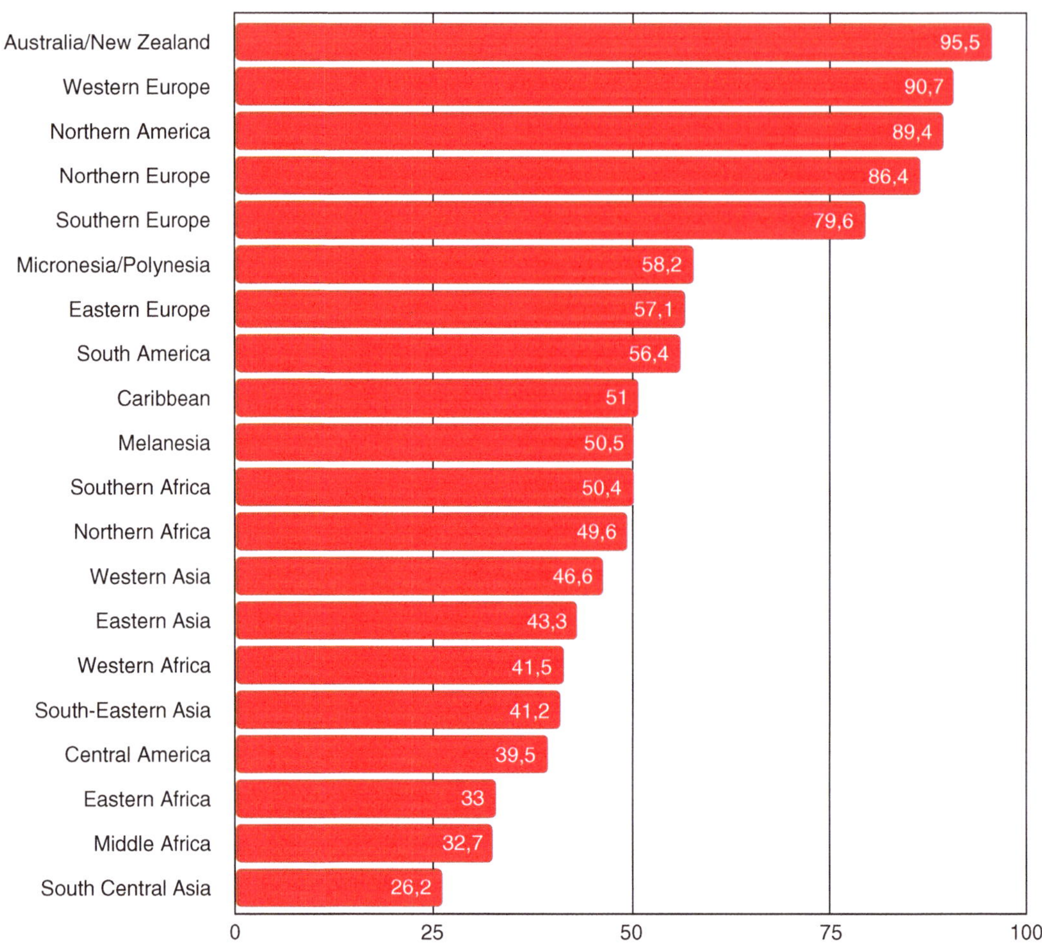

World Region-Specific Incidence Age-Standardised Rates for Female Breast Cancer in 2020 (Source; GLOBOSCAN 2020)

With a total of 523,000 estimated new cases in 2018 breast cancer is the leading female malignancy in Europe. Breast cancer accounts for the highest incidences in all European countries varying from 60 to 155 per 100,000. The most elevated rates are observed in Western Europe with the highest incidences for Benelux countries (Belgium, Luxembourg and The Netherlands) and in Northern Europe, particularly in the United Kingdom, Sweden and Finland. By contrast, breast cancer incidence rates are considerably lower in Eastern European countries. Breast cancer is also the leading cause of death in women constituting 16.2% of the total in Europe with 138,000 deceases. The highest mortality rates are seen in the Balkan Peninsula countries (Montenegro and Serbia, and Croatia) and in parts of Eastern Europe including Moldavia and Hungary. The lowest mortality rates are observed in South Europe (e.g. Spain and Portugal) and in the Nordic countries of Norway and Finland.

In the United States of America (USA), an estimated 268,600 new cases of invasive breast cancer diagnosed is expected for 2019. In addition, an estimated 48,100 cases of ductal carcinoma in situ (DCIS) will be diagnosed. Approximately 41,760 women are expected to die from breast cancer in 2019. More than 3.8 million women with a history of breast cancer in the USA were still alive on January 1, 2019. In this group, there are cancer-free patients and others who still had evidence of cancer and may have been undergoing treatment. More than 150,000 breast cancer survivors are living with metastatic disease, three-fourths of whom were originally diagnosed with stage I–III ([1–3]).

1.2 Breast Cancer Types and Subtypes

Globally, breast cancer can be divided into non-invasive or "in-situ" and invasive. Invasive breast cancer constitutes more than 80% of the cases and at present is considered a group of diseases with distinct histologic and molecular subtypes.

Non-invasive breast cancer has been historically divided into ductal carcinoma in situ (DCIS) and lobular carcinoma in situ (LCIS). LCIS is considered to be a benign condition associated with increased breast cancer risk but without the potential to progress to invasive cancer. Therefore, LCIS has been removed from the eighth AJCC breast cancer staging system. With respect to DCIS, it represents less than 20% of all breast cancer diagnoses and long-term studies have demonstrated that 20%–50% of patients with untreated DCIS are ultimately diagnosed with invasive breast cancer.

Size, shape and arrangement of breast cancer cells are important for histologic characterization of breast malignancies. More than 75% of invasive breast cancers are ductal carcinomas, now histologically categorized as "no special type". Invasive lobular carcinoma represents approximately 15% of invasive breast cancers. A wide variety of other rarer subtypes exist; for instance tubular, mucinous, cribriform and papillary carcinomas, which in general are associated with favourable prognoses. An uncommon but aggressive type is inflammatory breast cancer which is characterized by swelling and redness of the breast skin.

Breast cancer molecular subtypes are categorized according to the evaluation of biological markers like OR (Oestrogen Receptor), PR (Progesterone Receptor) and HER2 (Human epidermal growth factor type 2 receptor) and Ki67 protein. Hormone receptor positive (HR+) concerns those cancers that test positive for OR or PR, or both. Four principal subtypes are distinguished: Luminal A (HR+/HER2−/low Ki67), Luminal B (HR+/HER2±/high Ki67), Basal-like (HR-/HER2-) also called triple negative (OR-, PR- and HER2-), and HER2-enriched (HR-/HER2+).

Luminal A tumours are associated with a more favourable prognosis than Luminal B and triple-negative tumours. HER2-enriched tumours had the worst prognosis in the past but with the widespread use of targeted HER2+ therapies outcome has become significantly improved.

Luminal tumours are most common (60%–70%) and frequently presented as irregular masses without associated calcifications at mammography. Basal-like cancers (approximately 15% of all invasive breast cancers) are commonly presented as irregular tumours with ill-defined or spiculated margins although sometimes this type of tumours can be mistaken for benign lesions [1, 4, 5].

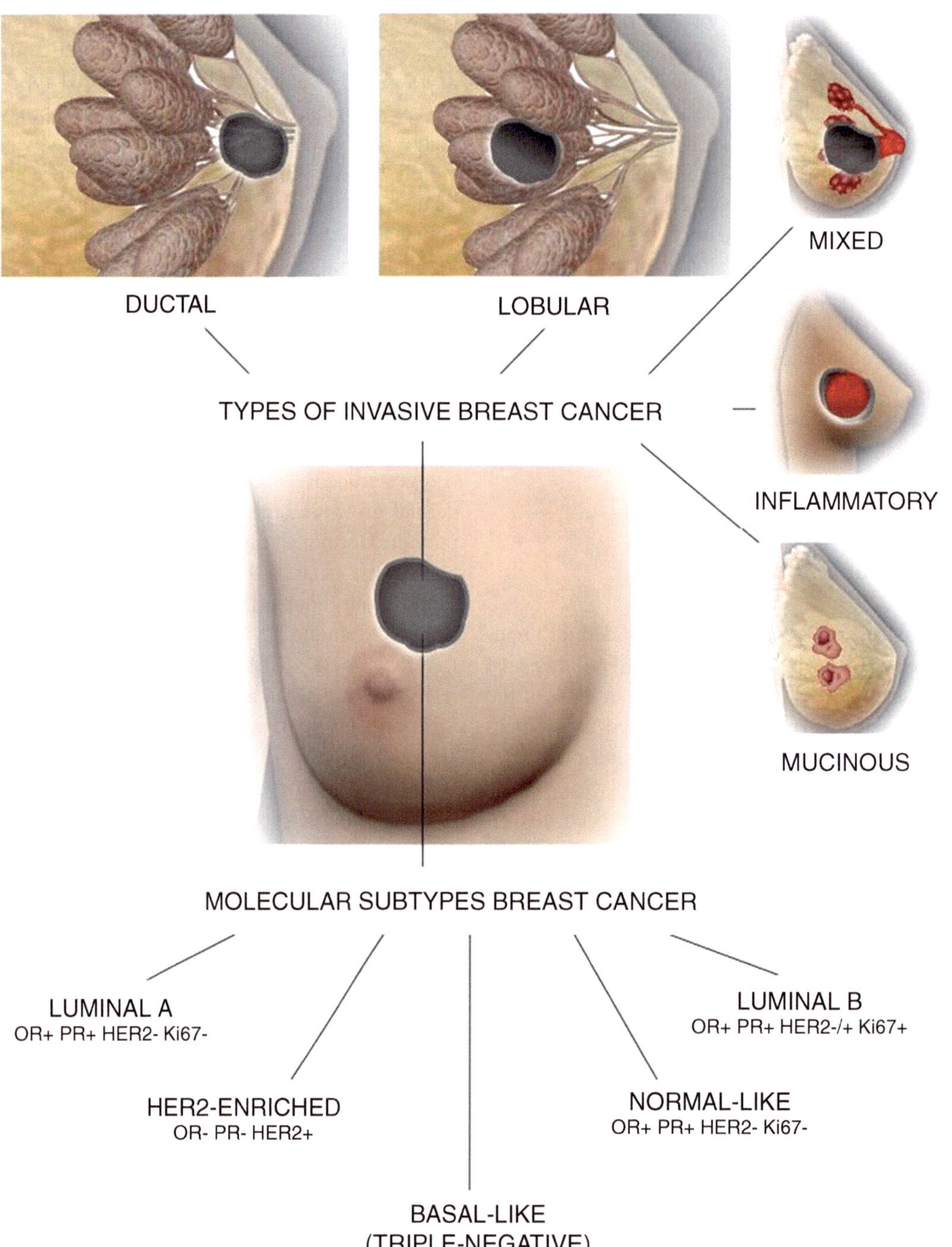
DUCTAL
LOBULAR
MIXED
TYPES OF INVASIVE BREAST CANCER
INFLAMMATORY
MUCINOUS
MOLECULAR SUBTYPES BREAST CANCER
LUMINAL A
OR+ PR+ HER2- Ki67-
LUMINAL B
OR+ PR+ HER2-/+ Ki67+
HER2-ENRICHED
OR- PR- HER2+
NORMAL-LIKE
OR+ PR+ HER2- Ki67-
BASAL-LIKE
(TRIPLE-NEGATIVE)
OR- PR- HER2- Basal Markers+

1.3 Breast Cancer Staging

The eighth edition of the TNM system for cancer staging of the UICC (Union for International Cancer Control) and AJCC (American Joint Committee on Cancer) was globally adopted on 01 January 2018.

With respect to primary tumour staging T1 disease is subcategorized as T1mi (tumour size ≤1 mm), T1a (>1 mm but ≤5 mm), T1b (>5 mm but ≤10 mm) and T1c (>10 mm but ≤20 mm). T2 concerns tumour size more than 20 mm but less or equal to 50 mm. T3 is related to tumours of more than 50 mm. T4 disease is subcategorized as T4a (thoracic wall invasion), T4b (macroscopic skin changes including ulceration and/or satellite skin nodules and/or edema) and T4d (inflammatory carcinoma). Thoracic wall invasion includes the ribs, intercostal muscles and serratus anterior muscle but not the pectoral muscles, which involvement does not affect T staging. At imaging, tumour size in at least the longest dimension should be measured to the nearest millimetre and in the case of discrepancies at mammography, ultrasound and/or MRI then MRI measurements are usually used.

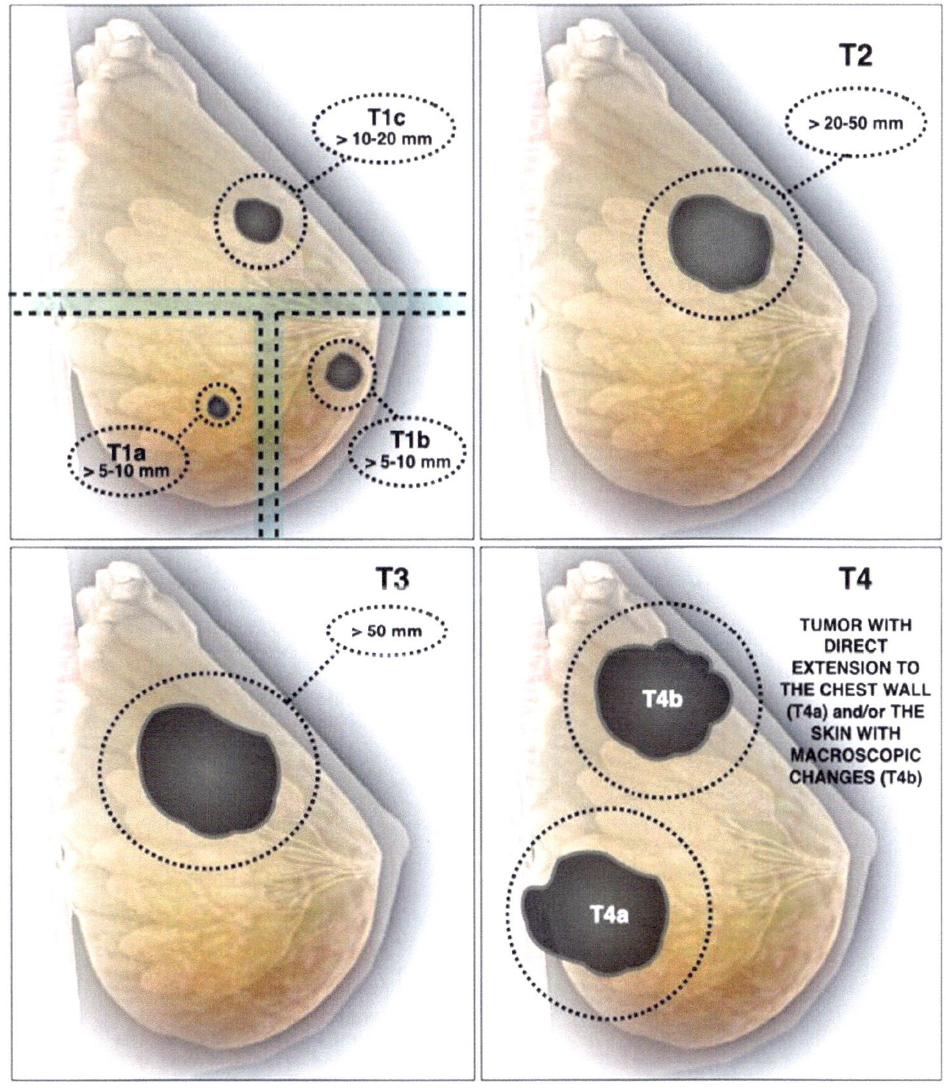

PRIMARY TUMOUR STAGING

For clinical regional staging both axillary and non-axillary (internal mammary, supraclavicular) lymph nodes are important. Axillary lymph nodes are divided in relation to the pectoralis minor muscle: level I concerns lymph nodes located lateral to its lateral border, level II those located between the lateral and medial borders including the interpectoral lymph nodes, and level III those located medial to medial border of the pectoral minor muscle and inferior to the clavicle. Staging cN0 concerns absent regional lymph node metastases. Category cN1 (metastases to movable ipsilateral level I and/or level II axillary nodes) includes cN1mi (micrometastases). Category cN2 disease includes cN2a (metastases to fixed or matted ipsilateral level I and/or level II axillary nodes), and cN2b (metastases to ipsilateral internal mammary nodes without axillary metastases. Category cN3 disease is subdivided into cN3a (metastases to ipsilateral level III axillary nodes with or without level I and/or level II axillary metastases), cN3b (metastases to ipsilateral internal mammary nodes with level I and/or level II axillary metastases) and cN3c (metastases to ipsilateral supraclavicular nodes). The ipsilateral supraclavicular nodal metastases are no longer considered stage IV disease in the eighth edition, because of the direct drainage of the upper inner portion of the breast to the supraclavicular lymph node group. By contrast, metastases to other lymph node groups like cervical lymph nodes, contralateral internal mammary lymph nodes or contralateral axillary lymph nodes are considered distant metastases.

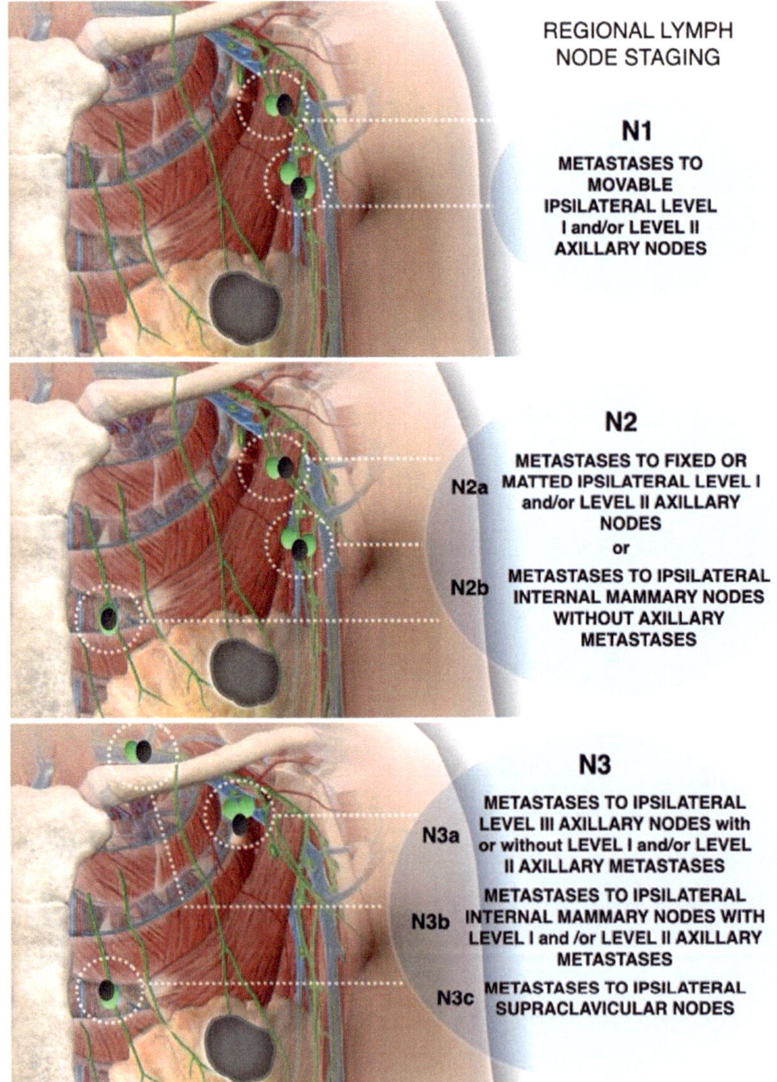

With respect to the quantity of lymph node metastases, the presence of any macroscopic lymph node metastasis indicates a minimum of stage II disease. N1 disease concerns 1–3 nodal metastases in level I and/or level II of the axilla whereas N2a disease involves 4–9 nodes in the same levels. N3 disease involves 10 or more nodes and indicates a minimum of stage IIIC disease.

Concerning distant metastases, the TNM classification recognizes the M0 category, which is associated with no clinical or imaging evidence of distant metastases, and M1 disease based on distant metastases evidenced by clinical or imaging findings. In the latter category metastases to the above-mentioned contralateral internal mammary and axillary lymph nodes as well as cervical lymph nodes are included. The four most common sites of distant metastases are bone, lung, brain, and liver. A subcategory of M0 concerns cM0(i+) for which tumour cells or deposits ≤0.2 mm have been detected in circulating blood, bone marrow or other nonregional nodal tissues but without clinical or imaging evidence of distant metastases.

The eighth edition of the TNM system for cancer staging contains four classification categories. The first category concerning clinical staging is designated by the prefix "c" and based on clinical examination, diagnostic imaging and core biopsy or aspiration sampling obtained prior to treatment. The second category receiving the prefix "p" concerns pathologic staging based on surgical specimens, including sentinel lymph node (SLN) biopsy. The third category designated by prefix "yp" applies to patients who have been treated with neoadjuvant therapy including chemotherapy, radiation or hormonal therapy. The last category applies to restaging in the presence of tumour recurrence.

Assessment of primary tumour size, regional lymphadenopathy and distant metastases results in an anatomic staging ranging from stage 0 (Tis, N0, M0) to stage IV (any T, any N, M1).

Although anatomic TNM classification remains the basis for the stage groups providing a common language for communication disease burden, the most significant adjustment in the eighth edition staging system is that final prognostic stage is determined by tumour histology (size, grade and presence of peritumoural vascular invasion), biomarker status (OR, PR, HER2), proliferation markers (e.g. Ki67), genomic panels and anatomic TNM stage. These additional determinants of outcome are now incorporated into parallel prognostic stage groups that recognize intrinsic tumour biology.

Gene expression profiles or multigene assays like MammaPrint, Oncotype DX Recurrence Score, Prosigna, Endopredict and Breast Cancer Index may be used to gain additional prognostic and/or predictive information to complement pathology assessment, to estimate risk and to predict the benefit of adjuvant chemotherapy [6–10].

1.4 Lymphatic Drainage of the Breast

Mammary lymphatic drainage is multidirectional. Drainage to the axilla is the principal lymphatic route. However, drainage to other lymph node groups like internal mammary, intramammary, interpectoral, periclavicular and paramammary nodal groups may also be observed. Most lymph from the breast flows to the nodal basins following a direct course, not passing through the subareolar plexus whose existence has not been demonstrated.

Caudally from the axillary vein, there are three levels of axillary lymph nodes (also known as Berg's levels) which are defined by their anatomic relationship to the pectoralis minor muscle. Level I concerns the nodal external mammary, lateral axillary vein, subscapular and axillary vein groups. The external mammary group, running parallel and along the lateral thoracic artery, primarily drains the lateral breast. The subscapular group, running parallel to the scapular vessels, drains the lower posterior neck, posterior trunk and posterior shoulder as well as the breast. The axillary vein group, located medial and posterior to the axillary veins, drains primarily from the upper extremity and not from the breast.

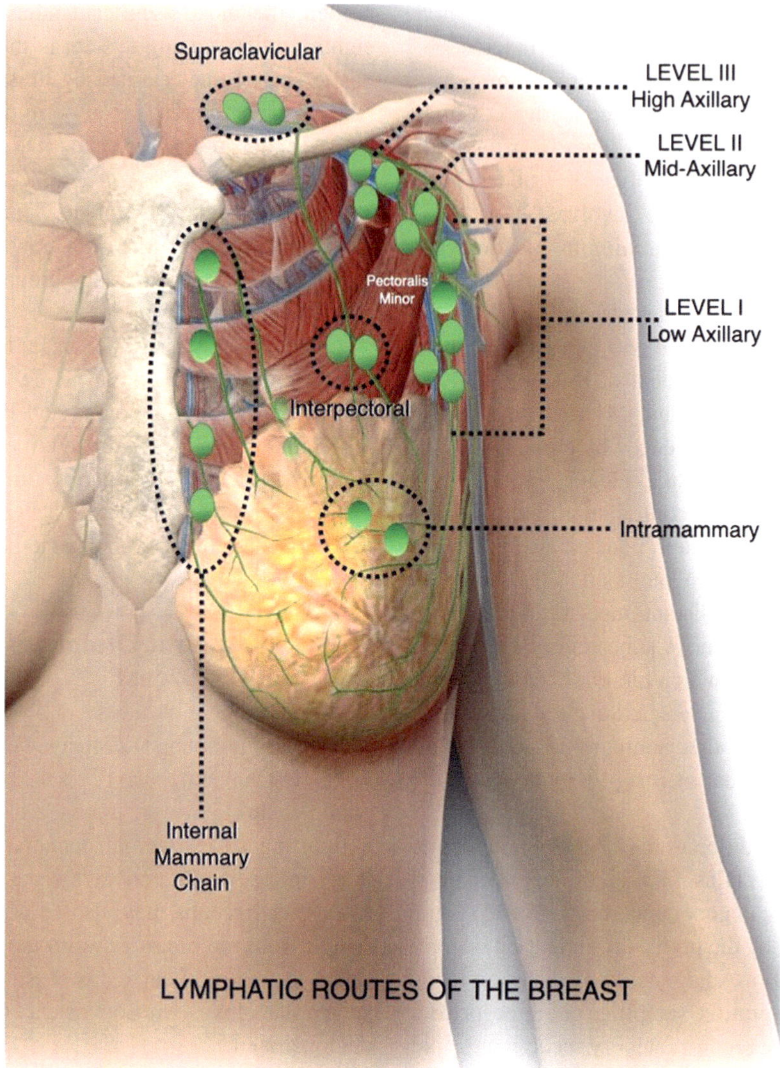

Lymph nodes of level II receive drainage directly from the breast but also from afferent vessels of level I lymph nodes. Most medial nodal groups of the axilla correspond to level III and drain from the other axillary groups but also merge with lymphatic vessels from the subclavicular group and the subclavian trunk. Some retromammary lymphatic vessels may penetrate the pectoralis major muscle and travelling along the thoracoacromial vessel, draining directly to level III. This level also may receive drainage from the superior and medial parts of the breast. Interpectoral lymph nodes located between the pectoralis muscles are also known as Rotter's nodes.

Besides the Berg's levels there is a more classical anatomical description that relates the axillary lymph node position to the anatomical limits of the axilla. This divides the axillary nodes into: (a) Anterior or antero-pectoral nodes, which are the nodes lying along the lateral border of pectoralis major near the lateral thoracic artery. (b) Posterior or subscapular nodes lying close to the posterior wall of the axilla near the subscapular artery. (c) Lateral nodes lying on the lateral wall of the axilla medial and posterior to the axillary vein. (d) Central nodes, lying at the mid base of the axilla in the axillary fat below or behind the pectoralis minor muscle. (e) Apical nodes, lying behind the upper part of pectoralis minor and extending above it. (f) Infraclavicular or subclavicular nodes, lying inferior to the clavicle above the apical nodes. (g) Interpectoral nodes, lying between the pectoralis major and pectoralis minor muscles.

With respect to the internal mammary chain these lymph nodes, particularly those nodes located in the first to fifth intercostal spaces, drain the posterocentral and posteromedial parts of the breast. Most internal mammary lymph nodes are located in the third intercostal space, then the second and the fourth with a tendency to encounter the nodes medial to the artery downwards from the second to the fourth spaces. Internal mammary lymph nodes are generally located in the intercostal spaces and the majority of retrocostal spaces do not contain any nodes [11–13].

1.5 The Sentinel Node Procedure

Due to its limited morbidity and high accuracy to identify axillary nodal metastases the sentinel node (SN) procedure has gradually replaced axillary lymph node dissection (ALND) in staging the axilla in patients with early breast cancer.

In breast cancer, the first applications of the procedure were based on the use of blue dye mapping, followed in 1993 by the incorporation of radiolabelled colloids for intraoperative radioguided detection using a gamma probe. Subsequently, mammary lymphoscintigraphy was added to the SN procedure based on its potential to map drainage patterns of individual breast cancers and to generate useful roadmaps to guide surgical SN biopsy.

The first indication for SN biopsy was established for T1 or T2 tumours without clinical evidence of axillary lymph node metastases and for more than 20 years these patients have constituted the primary source of clinical evaluation and long-term follow-up in many trials.

The clinical performance of radiocolloid-guided SN biopsy for these indications has been evaluated in a meta-analysis including 88 breast cancer studies resulting in a pooled SN identification rate of 94% increasing from 88% in the period 1992–2000 to 97% in the period 2007–2012 whereas the pooled false-negative rate was 2.2% in the whole period. This experience of almost 30 years has consolidated the role of radiocolloids to guide SN biopsy as the technique of choice and standard-of-care procedure.

SN biopsy may also be offered to patients who have operable breast cancer under the following circumstances: multicentric tumours (strength of recommendation: moderate), ductal carcinoma in situ (DCIS) when mastectomy will be performed (strength of recommendation: weak), prior breast and/or axillary surgery (strength of recommendation: strong), and preoperative neoadjuvant systemic therapy (strength of recommendation: moderate).

Due to insufficient data the SN procedure remains controversial for large or locally advanced invasive breast cancer (cT3 or cT4 tumours), inflammatory breast cancer, and DCIS when breast-conserving surgery is planned. According to more recent data SN biopsy can be omitted for this latter category.

In the last decade the introduction of neoadjuvant systemic treatment (NST) in patients with resectable early-stage breast cancer has become a standard of care facilitating the application of de-escalating surgery both in patients without axillary lymph node involvement and in patients with low-burden node-positive lymph node disease. In clinically negative axillary disease SN biopsy after NST is becoming accurate. In clinically positive axillary lymph nodes, the SN procedure is less accurate justifying its combination with marking of the affected axillary lymph nodes to accurately restage the axilla post-NST.

With the improvement of histopathology, due to the incorporation of immunohistochemistry (IHC) to the standard H&E (Haematoxylin & Eosin) examination, a significant increase in the detection of occult SN metastases has been possible. This has led to the incorporation of the categories of isolated tumour cells (<0.2 mm) and micrometastases (0.2–2 mm) to the TNM classification. Besides macrometastases (>2 mm) these occult metastases may be found in up to 16% of H&E negative SNs.

Treatment of the axilla has evolved from a dichotomized approach based on negative or positive SNs towards a more tailored axillary treatment based on the axillary tumour load. The non-inferiority in survival found for patients with tumour-negative SNs or with SN micrometastasis has led to consensus of performing SN biopsy alone as the standard management in these patients. By contrast, in patients with limited (one or two tumour-positive SNs) SN macrometastases, consensus is still lacking, although, due to the questions that arose about the necessity of ALND for these patients, there is a tendency to preserve the axilla.

Recent trial evaluation of patients with T1 or T2 invasive primary breast cancer and positive SNs has shown a comparable axillary control with locoregional radiotherapy in comparison with completion ALND. Other prospective trials have revealed that a 10-year overall survival for patients treated with SN biopsy alone is not inferior to those treated with completion ALND.

In recent studies, patients with internal mammary metastatic SNs were found to have worse survival due to distant metastases with a higher incidence associated to tumours larger than 1.5 cm. Therefore, surgical removal of internal mammary SNs, if technically possible, from patients younger than 70 years with tumours larger than 1.5 cm, can be considered. This approach, which may affect clinical management regarding not only locoregional treatment, but also systemic therapy, revalues lymphoscintigraphy by means of tumour-related injections which is the only modality able to depict parasternal drainage [14–18].

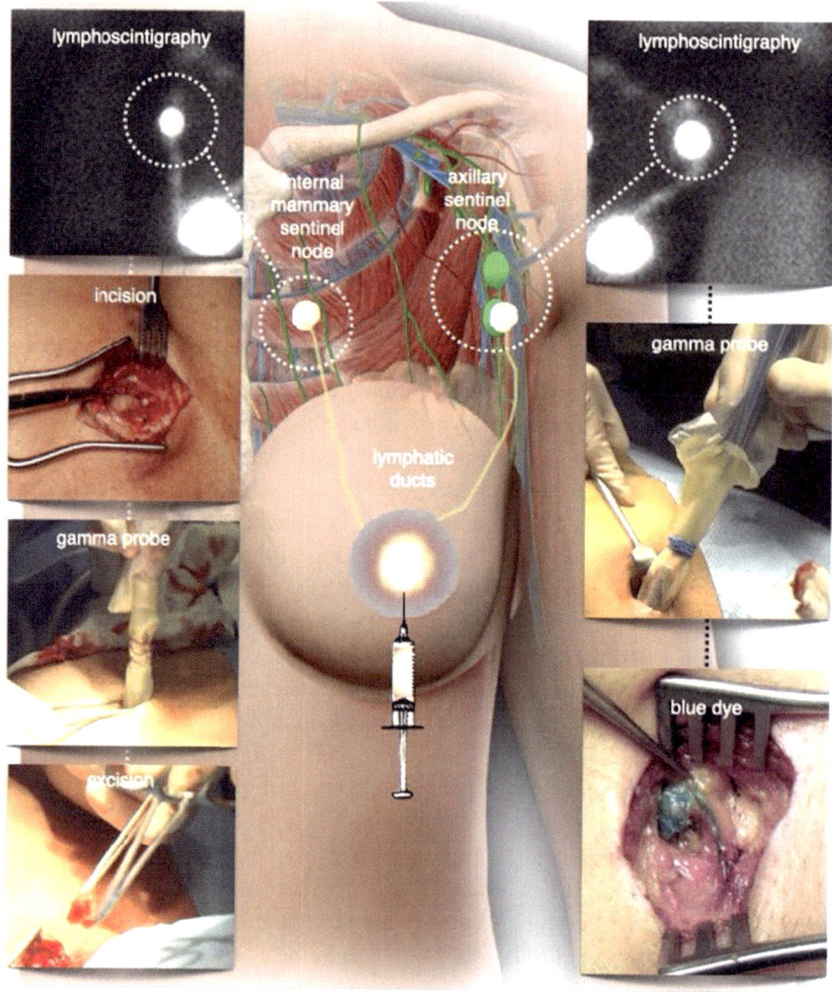

The
SENTINEL NODE PROCEDURE
axillary & non-axillary drainage

1.6 Preoperative Sentinel Node Lymphoscintigraphy and SPECT/CT

With some particular recommendations, the protocol of mammary lymphoscintigraphy is comparable with the image acquisition of other SN procedures.

For mammary lymphoscintigraphy dynamic imaging is not mandatory and is frequently replaced by early static planar images acquired 10–20 min after radiotracer administration using a LVOF gamma camera in order to depict the pattern of the entire draining lymphatic basins in a single image.

Delayed images are recommended to be acquired 2–4 h after radiocolloid injection. At each acquisition time at least two, and preferably three, 5-min images are recommended: anterior, lateral and 45° anterior oblique. Anterior images are acquired with the patient lying supine with the arm extended perpendicular to the body. Lateral images are acquired in the same position with the arm of the affected side in extension. Alternatively, for lateral views the patient may be rotated 90° lying on the contralateral side to facilitate positioning of the camera on the affected side. Also, rotation to a prone position ("hanging breast" position) with the gamma camera vertically positioned from lateral to the affected side in order to increase the distance between the injection and the SNs is possible. For the 45° anterior oblique images the patient preferentially needs to rotate from supine to 45° with the arm positioned above the head.

Simultaneously acquired transmission images using a ^{57}Co or ^{99m}Tc flood source positioned under the patient's trunk, opposite the camera detector, help to delineate contour of the breast and axillary areas. Based on the findings of lymphoscintigraphy the exact position of the SN is marked with indelible ink on the skin with the aid of a radioactive point source and real time gamma camera imaging. The marking process needs to be performed with the arm at an abduction of about 90°, approximately the same position of the patient during surgery. Skin marking can also be assisted by the gamma probe using external counting.

With the integration of a fast high-end CT component to modern LVOF dual-head gamma cameras SPECT/CT can be acquired in the same session as planar lymphoscintigraphy. SPECT/CT depicts SNs in an anatomical environment with the possibility to accurately indicate their location in relation to pectoral muscles, blood vessels, lymph node groups, surgical axillary levels and intercostal spaces.

SPECT/CT fusion images can be displayed in relation to the CT component following multiple reconstruction (MPR) and the use of cross-reference lines allows the navigation between axial, coronal and sagittal views. For fused images the anatomical CT information is displayed as background using a grey scale, whereas SPECT serves as foreground image displaying SN uptake with a colour scale.

Because of its higher spatial resolution, SPECT/CT detects more SNs than planar imaging and also changes the information concerning drainage territory in almost 20% of the patients.

SPECT/CT indications for SN in breast cancer can be summarized as follows:

(a) To visualize SNs in case of non-visualization on planar images; for instance in patient obesity. This is possible due to the SPECT/CT correction for attenuation and scatter.
(b) To identify SNs in cases with inconclusive planar images, e.g. SNs located close to the injection site, suspicion of skin contamination and SN localization in uncommon axillary and non-axillary sites.
(c) To localize SNs in patients with ipsilateral cancer relapse after treatment with breast surgery or radiotherapy in the past. For this group SPECT/CT is mandatory due to a higher SN visualization and a 60% territory mismatch between planar images and SPECT/CT [19–21].

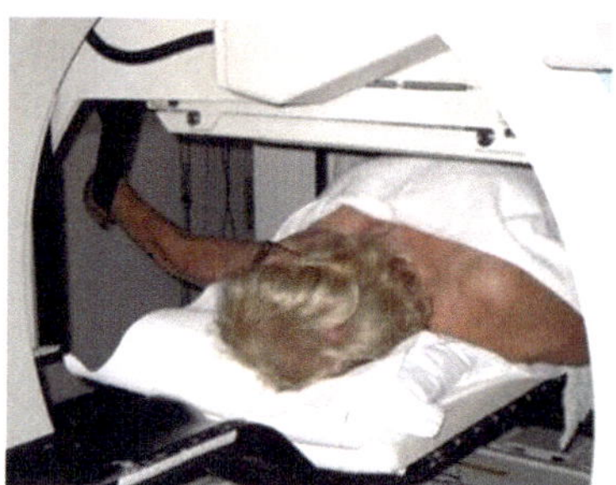

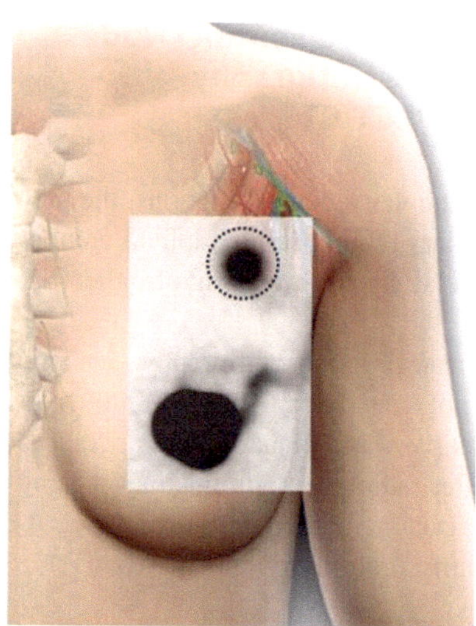

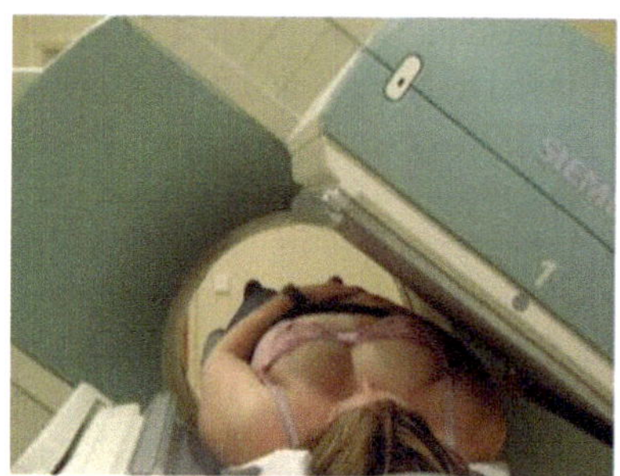

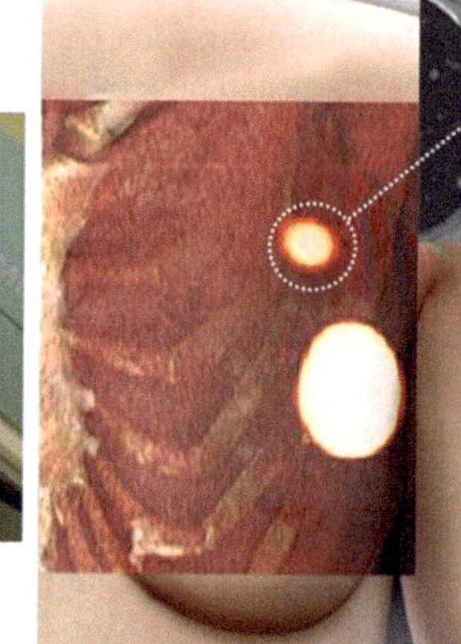

1.7 Radiotracer Administration for Sentinel Node Mapping

There is no consensus on optimal injection technique for breast cancer. First validation studies concerned deep tumour-related injections (intratumoural or peritumoural).

Peritumoural administration for mammary lymphoscintigraphy was introduced in the early period of the SN procedure on the basis of four small volume injections around the tumour and became one of the most used techniques to combine preoperative lymphatic mapping and intraoperative SN detection in later years. Intratumoural administration is based on a single small volume injection and is probably the technique with the highest reproducibility.

Deep injections can be performed guided by palpation or ultrasound when tumours are not palpable. For this latter category single intratumoural administration guided by ultrasound or stereotaxis can facilitate the combination of SN biopsy and occult lesion localization (SNOLL) in the same intraoperative session when a radiocolloid appropriate for both tumour retention and migration to lymph nodes is used.

Superficial radiocolloid administration includes intradermal, subcutaneous, subareolar and periareolar injection techniques. These techniques are independent of the palpable or nonpalpable nature of the tumour and have gained in popularity in recent years principally due to their high practicability with minimum training and high SN detection in the axilla.

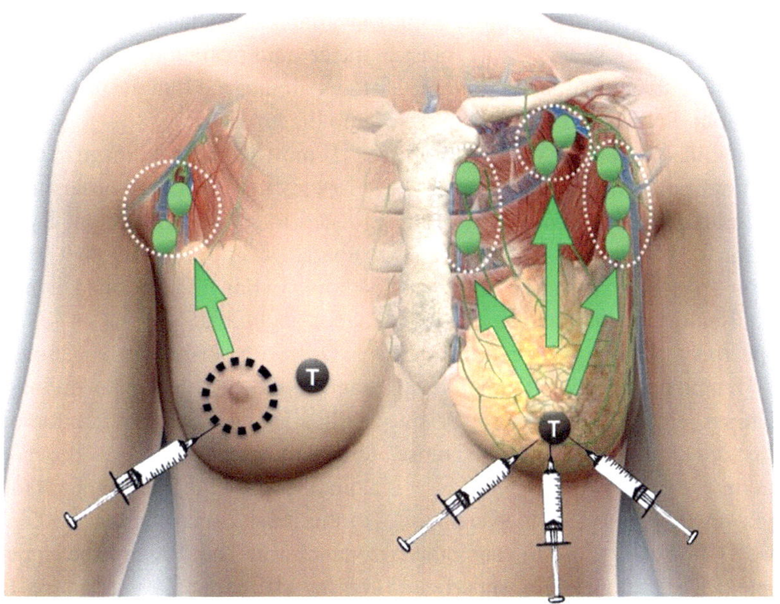

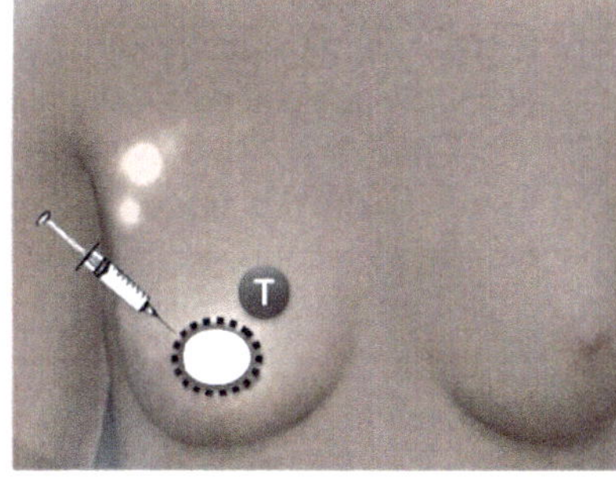

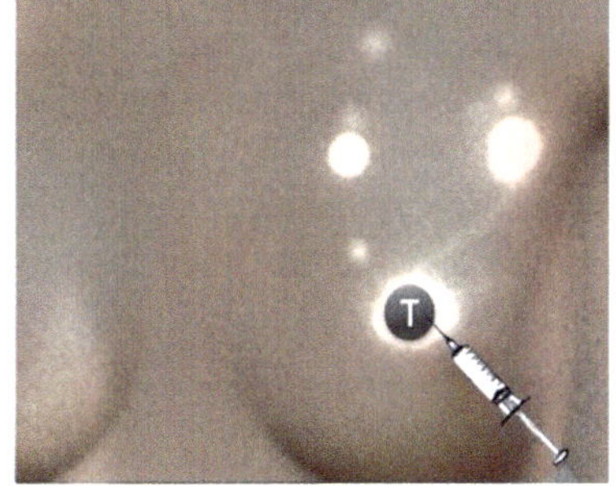

Despite this variability in various meta-analyses, no significant differences between deep and superficial radiotracer injections for axillary SN identification on lymphoscintigraphy or during surgery have been found; by contrast, the rate of extra-axillary SN identification is significantly higher when deep, rather than superficial, injection is used.

Recent insights support the approach that the choice for an optimal injection approach will depend on the specific clinical indications. Superficial injections may be adequate for patients with low risk for SN metastases like small or superficially located tumours in the upper lateral quadrant of the breast where the purpose is to spare an unnecessary ALND. In high-risk patients with large or multifocal tumours, or tumours located deep or medio-caudally in the breast wherein accurate staging including SNs outside the axilla is wanted, a deep tumour-related injection technique appears to be more appropriate.

A tracer administration approach combining deep and superficial injections to facilitate both improved SN detection and decreased false-negative results, is increasingly recommended in recent years. A triple-site radiotracer injection is associated with a 98% SN visualization rate.

Non-visualization has been associated with factors such as age (≥70 years), body mass index (≥30 kg/m^2) and nonpalpable tumours. In patients without SN visualization reinjection of radiocolloids increases visualization. Also the combination of deep and superficial injections simultaneously may prevent non-visualization.

Major criteria for SN identification are determined by the visualization of lymphatic ducts, the time of appearance, the lymph node basin and the intensity of lymph node uptake. In mammary lymphoscintigraphy either by superficial or by deep tracer injection axillary drainage is the most occurring pattern.

Frequently a single axillary SN is visualized. Less often two SNs, usually close to each other, may be depicted. The rationale for superficial radiocolloid administration is based on the assumption that draining axillary SN should invariably lie in the anterior lymph node groups of level I.

In topographic studies using subareolar injection SNs in the antero-pectoral group have been found in 68% and in the mid nodal group in 38% of the patients. However, when deep injections around the tumour site in the breast are administered, drainage to level I (89%), level II (9%) and level III (2%) occurs whereas about 50% of SNs in level I of the axilla is located outside the anterior group of nodes.

Different from the axillary drainage the visualization of SNs outside the axilla is almost invariably associated with deep tumour-related tracer administration, either by multiple injections around the tumour or by a single injection into the tumour.

From 15 to 30% drainage to the internal mammary chain (IMC) is observed after tumour-related tracer administration. By contrast, when subareolar injection or other superficial tracer administration is performed non-axillary drainage is negligible.

Deep tumour-related injections in any quadrant of the breast lead to drainage outside the axilla. Using a single intratumoural injection drainage to the IMC was observed in 52% of tumours in the inner lower quadrant, 32% located in the inner upper quadrant, 30% located in the outer lower and 10% in the upper outer quadrants, whereas a 24% drainage from centrally located tumours occurred.

When drainage to the IMC occurs, 87% SNs are found in the second, third and fourth intercostal spaces. Besides IMC drainage SNs may also be found in intramammary, interpectoral, periclavicular and paramammary locations.

When the breast has been treated (surgery, adjuvant systemic treatment, radiotherapy) there is less ipsilateral axillary drainage (70%) and an increased incidence of aberrant lymphatic drainage with a total of 51% drainage outside the ipsilateral axilla. This includes IMC (31%), interpectoral (7%), intramammary (6%), periclavicular (3.5%) and contralateral axilla (3.5%) [13, 22–26].

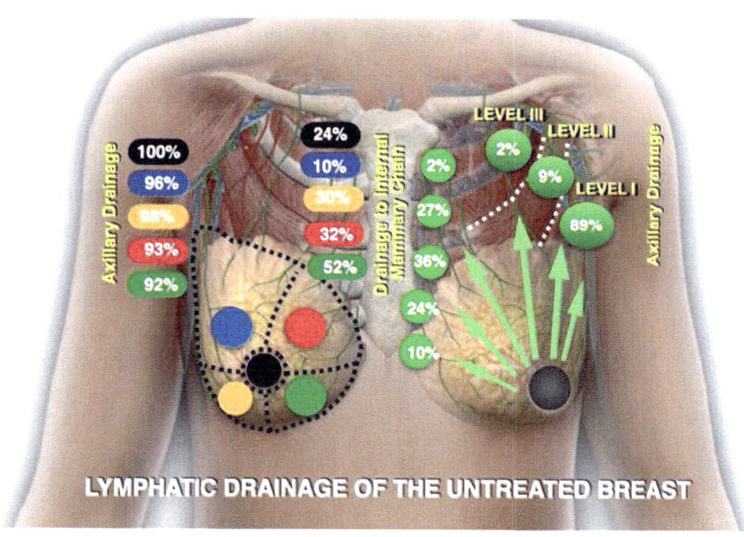
Axillary Drainage
100%
96%
98%
93%
92%
24%
10%
30%
32%
52%
Drainage to Internal Mammary Chain
2%
27%
36%
24%
10%
LEVEL III
2%
LEVEL II
9%
LEVEL I
89%
Axillary Drainage
LYMPHATIC DRAINAGE OF THE UNTREATED BREAST

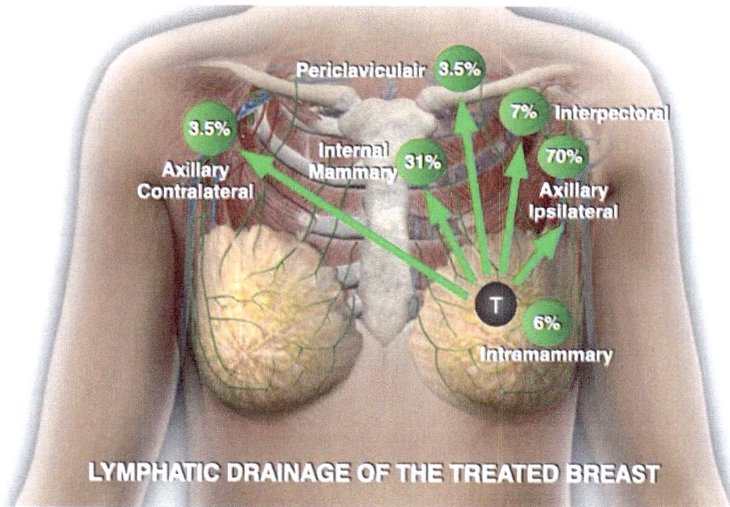
Periclaviculair 3.5%
7% Interpectoral
3.5%
Axillary Contralateral
Internal Mammary
31%
70%
Axillary Ipsilateral
T
6%
Intramammary
LYMPHATIC DRAINAGE OF THE TREATED BREAST

1.8 Intraoperative Sentinel Node Detection

For intraoperative SN detection, the most used device is the gamma probe which enables to count radioactivity in the surgical field providing a numerical readout and audible signals proportional to the counting rate.

Commercially available gamma probes can be divided into crystal scintillation and semiconductor probes. Independent of the type, the energy window for detection/counting is set on the 140-keV peak of ^{99m}Tc. Probes need to combine an adequate sensitivity to detect weakly active SNs (e.g. due to low nodal uptake or by soft tissue attenuation when nodal uptake is measured from the skin surface) with enough power to discriminate activity within a SN which requires a well-collimated probe for a small angle view.

Gamma probes are cylindrical with diameters varying from 10 to 18 mm. Some models are slightly angled to facilitate handling in the surgical field. Wired probe needs to be connected through flexible cables with sterilized wrapping to small control units, usually equipped with a portable laptop or tablet. In the last decade, wireless Bluetooth-based probes have become available; the most recent introduced models are made of metal that can be sterilized.

In the operating room, the skin marking indicated by the nuclear physician during gamma camera imaging is used by the surgeon as orientation for the incision which is performed at the site with highest counts assisted with a gamma probe. Subsequently, the gamma probe is introduced through the skin incision to localize the radioactive SN, which is generally easily identified by acoustic signals emitted from the control unit. Localization can be combined with the use of blue dye injected 10–20 min before the surgical act. After SN excision, the operative field is controlled for residual activity with the gamma probe. Counting per unit time is recorded in the operative field over the SN before and after excision.

In non-axillary SN biopsy gamma probe counting is the most important aspect. Blue dyes are not helpful due to their lack of migration to lymph node basins outside the axilla. In these cases, the additional use of a portable gamma camera (PGC) may enhance the reliability of the SN procedure by providing high-resolution SN imaging. These devices are also helpful in cases with axillary drainage in the vicinity of the injection site. Due to their visualization on-screen SN images after excision can be compared with those before excision. Residual focal activity at the same location is usually associated with a second SN.

In recent years more sophisticated gamma-based devices have incorporated freehandSPECT technology for three-dimensional imaging of the axillary SN radiotracer distribution in breast cancer patients by tracking the location of the gamma probes or portable cameras [27, 28].

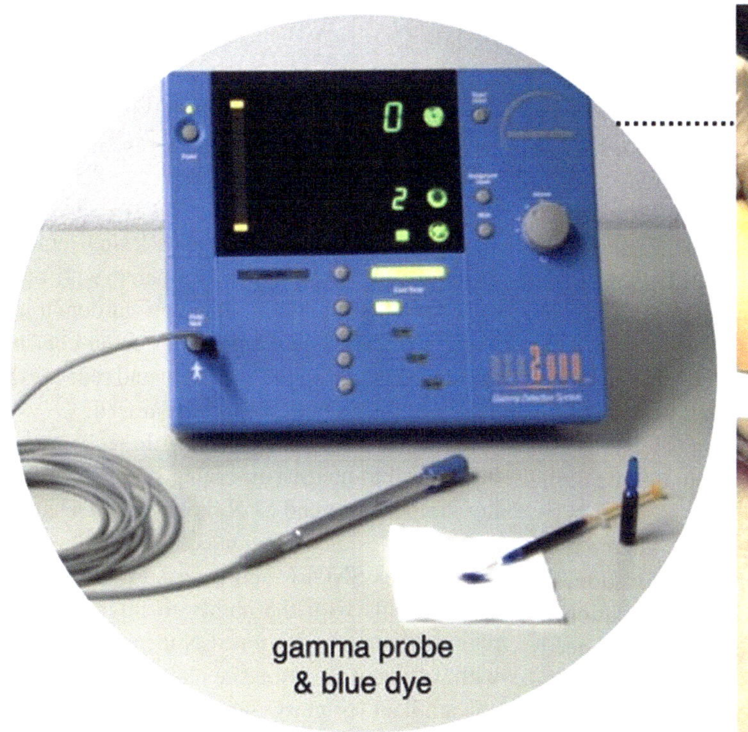
gamma probe
& blue dye

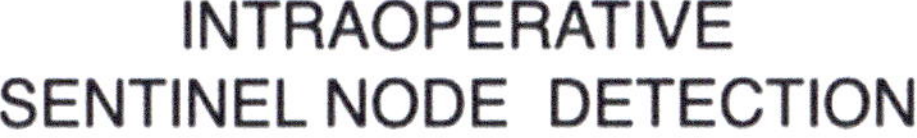
INTRAOPERATIVE
SENTINEL NODE DETECTION

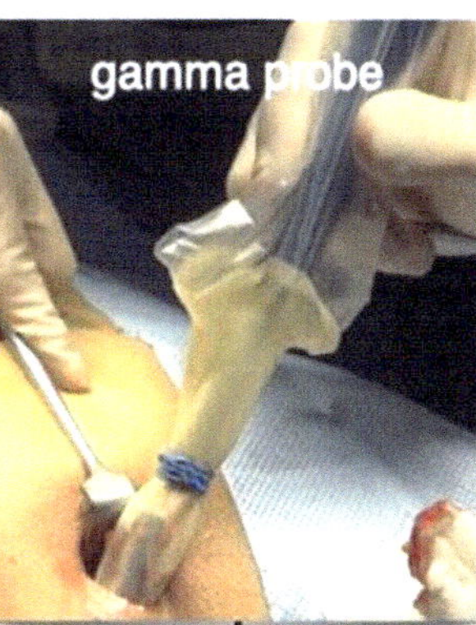
gamma probe

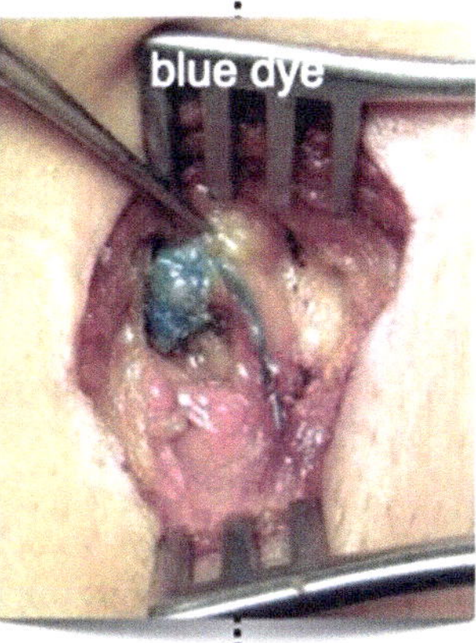
blue dye

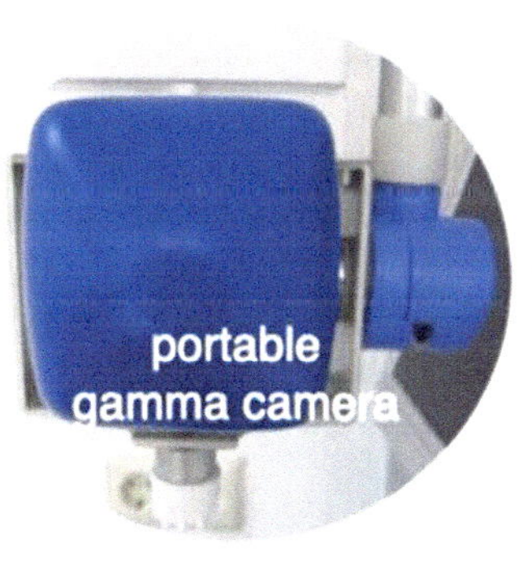
portable
gamma camera

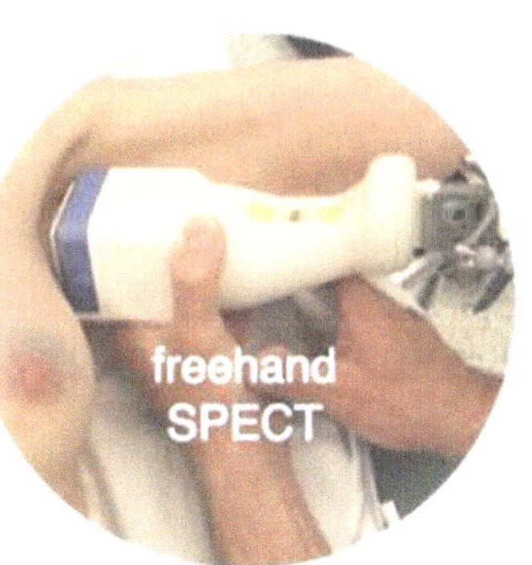
freehand
SPECT

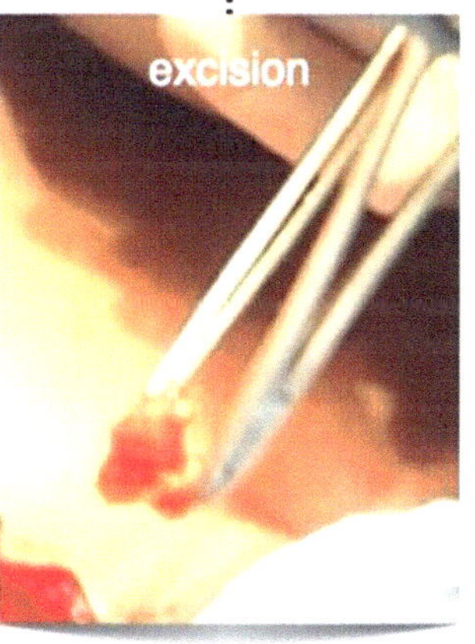
excision

1.9 Radioguided Occult Lesion Localization

Intralesional tracer administration enabling excisional biopsy of primary breast lesions is an application known as ROLL (Radioguided Occult Lesion Localization).

The first clinical validation of Radioguided Occult Lesion Localization (ROLL) was based on a direct intralesional injection of macroaggregates of albumin (MAA) labelled with ^{99m}Tc in nonpalpable breast lesions guided by ultrasonography or stereotactic mammography. ^{99m}Tc-MAA with a particle size of 10–150 μm is retained into the tumour without migration from the site of the injection.

ROLL can be performed on the same day or on the next day after tracer administration. To accomplish concentricity in the distribution of the tracer into the tumour the radiotracer needs to be injected as centrally as possible in the lesion. At the operating room, skin incision is guided by a gamma probe after searching for the site with highest counts or at a site suitable for oncoplastic breast surgery. During excision, the gamma probe is introduced through a small skin incision that can ensure an optimal cosmetic outcome without the topographic constraints required by the classical intralesional markers. Intraoperative gamma probe counting enables the surgeon to easily localize the focal deposition of ^{99m}Tc-MAA, thereby facilitating the procedure.

After lesion removal residual activity in the surgical field must be checked to avoid the possibility of missing some residual involved tissue.

The surgical specimen is checked ex vivo with the gamma probe for further confirmation of radioactivity, and can also be X-rayed to ensure complete removal of the area containing the lesion.

The ROLL technique enables lesion removal in almost all cases. When compared with other localization techniques including carbon tracer and hooked wire, ROLL provides better centring of the lesion within the specimen and reduces the amount of healthy tissue to be removed.

Since a few years, the ROLL technique is being used in breast-conserving surgery combining lumpectomy and SLN biopsy by means of a single intralesional tracer injection. This approach is known as SNOLL and is based on the use of radiocolloids with the ability to migrate to the regional lymph nodes for SLN identification, but with sufficient injection site retention to facilitate concomitant primary tumour resection. Basic work based on ex vivo lymph node measurements demonstrated that when ^{99m}Tc-nanocolloid is administered into a breast tumour, only 2–3% migrate to the axillary SLNs.

Devices such as portable gamma cameras and freehand SPECT are useful not only to guide tumour excision but also to control for concentricity of the radioactive lesion in relation to the specimen margins. Freehand SPECT can facilitate 3D margin analysis whereas a new generation of portable gamma cameras with embedded optical camera support can display the lesion within the specimen [29, 30].

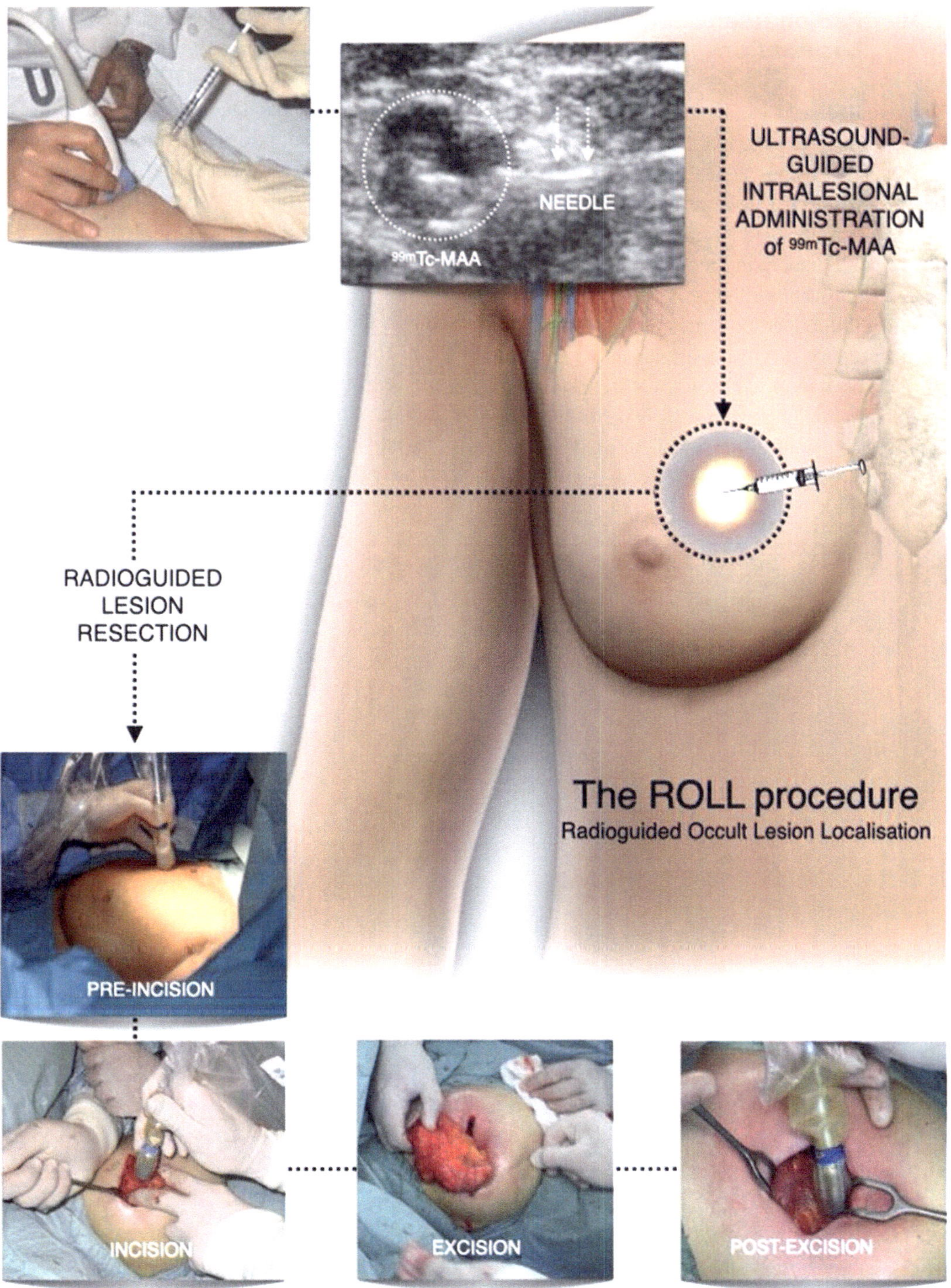
NEEDLE
^{99m}Tc-MAA
ULTRASOUND-GUIDED INTRALESIONAL ADMINISTRATION of ^{99m}Tc-MAA
RADIOGUIDED LESION RESECTION
The ROLL procedure
Radioguided Occult Lesion Localisation
PRE-INCISION
INCISION
EXCISION
POST-EXCISION

1.10 Radioguided Seed Localization

Radioguided seed localization (RSL) was introduced a few years ago to guide excision of breast lesions. RSL, using ^{125}I-seeds, appears to be comparable with ROLL with respect to outcome and is based on the use of similar gamma probe devices in the operating room.

No significant differences concerning specimen weight, reoperation rates and five-year local recurrence-free survival in impalpable breast cancer have been reported between RSL and ROLL.

Reoperation rate using RSL is better than procedures using hooked wire localization. Therefore, RSL is considered to be cost-effective.

With respect to locally advanced breast cancer receiving neoadjuvant chemotherapy, RSL is also comparable with ROLL but with more practical advantages. Due to the long half-life of ^{125}I, seed implantation to guide excision of residual tumour may occur before chemotherapy without additional tracer injection, as is necessary for ROLL, after completing neoadjuvant treatment.

The ^{125}I-seeds (<8Mbq) are essentially the same as the ones used for brachytherapy of cancer of the prostate, namely, a 4.5–0.8 mm titanium capsule containing a ceramic cylinder enriched with ^{125}I-iodine, which has a long decay time (half-life of 59.4 days) and emits low-energy photons (27 keV).

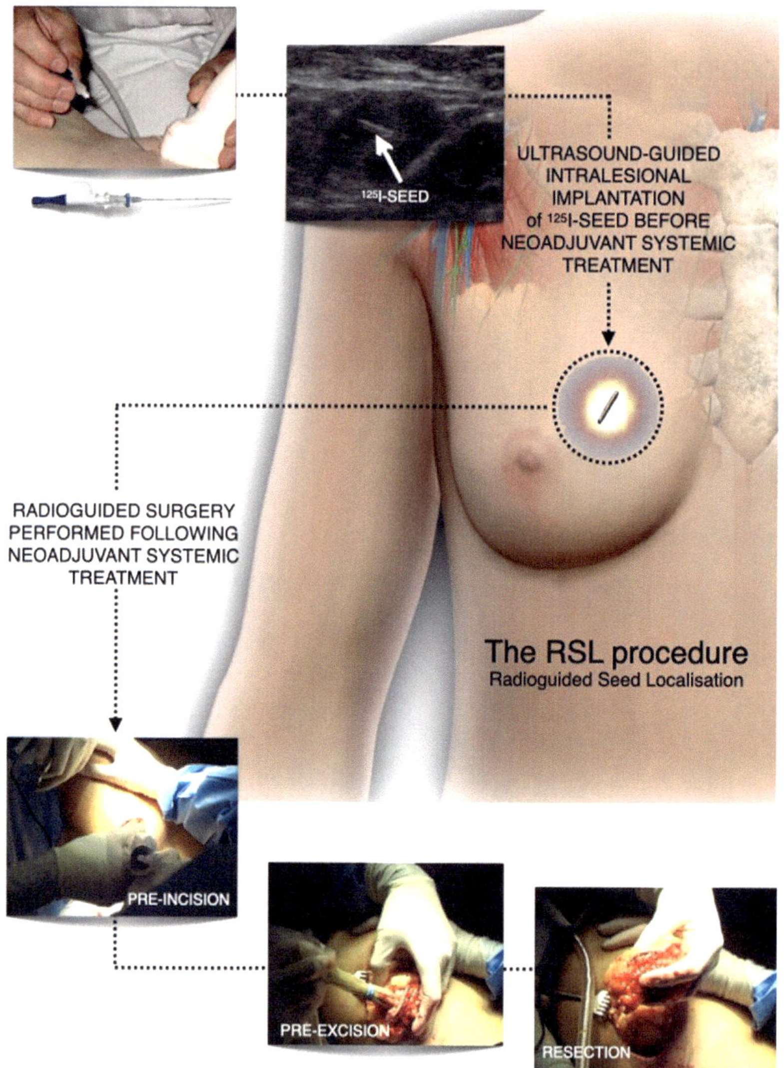

The use of one ^{125}I-seed with this low photon energy has a negligible effect on the surrounding tissue. The radioactive seed is placed, under mammographic or ultrasonographic guidance, in the centre of the breast lesion using an 18-G needle fixed in a needle holder; after successful positioning the exact location is confirmed by mammography.

During surgery excision of the lesion is guided by using a handheld gamma probe. Following transcutaneous measurements with this gamma probe the site of the maximum counts is determined and its location is marked on the skin to guide incision by the surgeon. Subsequently, excision of the tumour containing the radioactive seed is effectuated. Correct excision is confirmed by measurements indicating absence of ^{125}I signals in the wound accompanied by positive counting in the excised specimen.

In a similar manner as for ROLL, devices like freehand SPECT and portable gamma cameras can be useful to implement RSL with a more accurate approach incorporating images to guide excision and to check margin assessment [31–34].

1.11 Targeted Lymph Node Biopsy: The MARI Procedure

The procedure known as MARI (Marking Axillary lymph nodes with Radioactive Iodine seeds) is based on the implantation of ^{125}I-seeds in axillary metastatic lymph nodes before neoadjuvant chemotherapy.

Radioactive seeds are associated with a decreased risk for displacement in the time between insertion and surgery. Therefore, risk of injury to vascular structures in the surrounding area is negligible.

Prior to seed insertion fine-needle aspiration biopsy is required to determine the intended lymph node. Usually a single lymph node (typically the largest is selected for biopsy and seed insertion although in cases with multiple nodal disease more lymph nodes may be selected.

The ^{125}I-seed is placed within an 18-G needle after occluding its tip with sterile bone wax. The positive lymph node is visualized by ultrasonography and a small incision is made in the skin under local anaesthesia. Subsequently, the needle tip is guided to the lymph node and a stylet is used to displace the radioactive seed through the bone wax and into the node. After the needle is withdrawn the position of the seed is confirmed by ultrasonography and a gamma probe. The procedure is usually combined with marking of the primary tumour (RSL).

Following completion of neoadjuvant chemotherapy removal of the marked lymph node is undertaken mostly in the same session as RSL of the primary lesion. Using the gamma probe the point of the highest activity over the surface of the axilla is determined and subsequently marked on the skin with ink. Excision of the marked node is assisted with the gamma probe and after removal the axilla is checked to assess absence of radiation. The removed MARI node is then stored in a lead container and transported to the pathology department.

For histopathology the marked node is bisected and completely embedded in paraffin. Blocks are cut at three levels with a minimum of 150 um intervals. The pathologist extracts the seed from the lymph node specimen under guidance of the gamma probe and after storage in a lead container it is transported to a storage facility for decay.

The MARI procedure is recognized in the literature as one of the modalities of Targeted Lymph Node Biopsy (TLNB) which includes the selective removal of metastatic lymph node(s) marked before neoadjuvant therapy. The combination of TNLB with SN biopsy is known as Targeted Axillary Dissection (TAD).

MARI is able to reach a 97% lymph node identification rate with an acceptable false-negative rate (7%) in predicting complete response in the affected axilla. No relevant loss of ^{125}I-signal is observed during 17–18 weeks. The high success rate of MARI is based on the detection of the radioactive signals with the gamma probe. This is a major technical advantage in comparison with the use of lost clips which can only be removed using guidance by radiography, ultrasound or computer tomography.

When TAD (MARI + SN biopsy) is performed the success rate is almost similar (>98%) as with MARI alone but false-negative rate tends to be lower (2–4%).

Although MARI and TAD appear to be successful there is no consensus concerning the number of lymph nodes that should be marked in patients with more than one suspicious lymph node on imaging (ultrasound, ^{18}F-FDG PET/CT). Marking of a single node has as advantages a lower cost, possibly less arm morbidity (fewer nodes are removed) and an easier marking procedure. Marking of all suspicious nodes is potentially associated to lower false-negative rates but it may lead to higher costs, higher probability that one of the marked nodes is not removed, more arm morbidity and a complicated marking procedure [35–38].

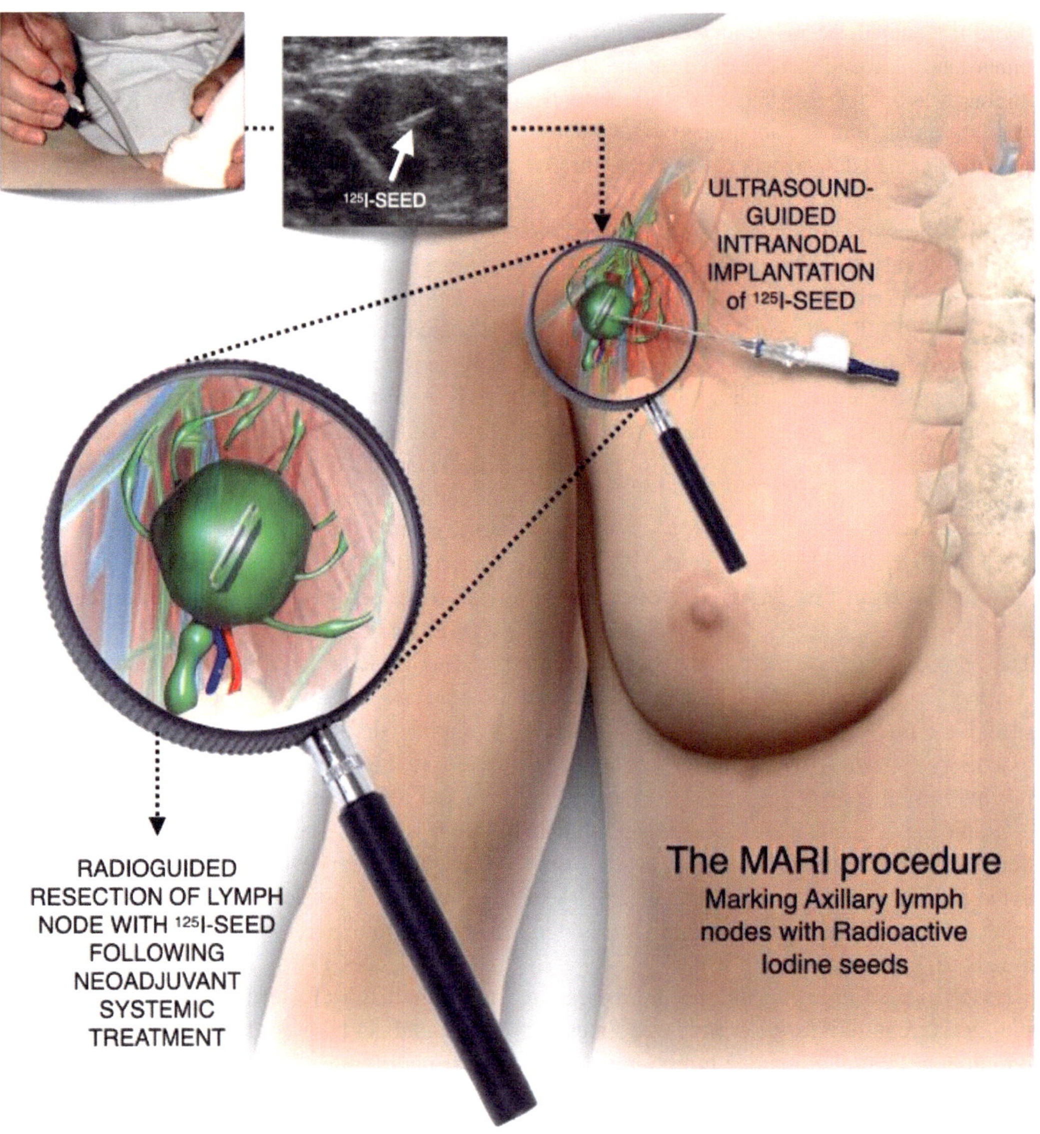

1.12 ^{18}F-FDG and Breast Cancer

^{18}F-FDG uptake in breast cancer is influenced by its histologic type, receptor status and malignancy grade.

Considering histological subtypes, IDC tumours, which account for 75–80% of primary breast cancers, have higher ^{18}F-FDG avidity than ILC, which account for 10–15% of breast lesions. This aspect is not only related to primary tumour but also to metastases. Untreated bone metastases from ILC are more frequently missed than IDC metastases because their avidity is often not higher than the background. Another factor is that the pattern of spread of ILC recognizes a greater propensity to metastasize to the gastrointestinal tract and retroperitoneum which are areas with common accumulation of ^{18}F-FDG. This is one of the reasons explaining the lower detection rates of PET/CT for distant metastases of ILC in comparison to IDC. Careful reading of the associated CT is therefore of extra importance.

Concerning hormone receptor status, FDG uptake is lower in well-differentiated OR-positive tumours than OR-negative tumours. The same pattern is observed for PR-positive tumours which show less ^{18}F-FDG avidity than PR-negative malignancies.

With respect to tumour phenotype triple-negative tumours, i.e. OR negative, PR negative and having no over expression of HER2 (ERBB2) show substantially higher FDG avidity than other tumours. Among luminal tumours, FDG uptake is lower in luminal A than in luminal B.

Breast cancer grade is also of influence in the avidity of ^{18}F-FDG. The higher the grade the higher the uptake. Grade 1 or 2 tumours are less avid than grade 3 lesions. Grades 1, 2 and 3 are also named "well differentiated", "moderately differentiated" and "poorly differentiated", respectively.

With respect to proliferation index, FDG uptake is weaker in low-proliferative tumours as assessed by the Ki67 index.

Based on available data ^{18}F-FDG PET/CT is certainly helpful (use recommended) for staging from clinical stage IIB and possibly helpful (use optional) in stage IIA (T1N1 or T2N0) but it does not offer added value (use not recommended) in stage I (T1N0) [39–41].

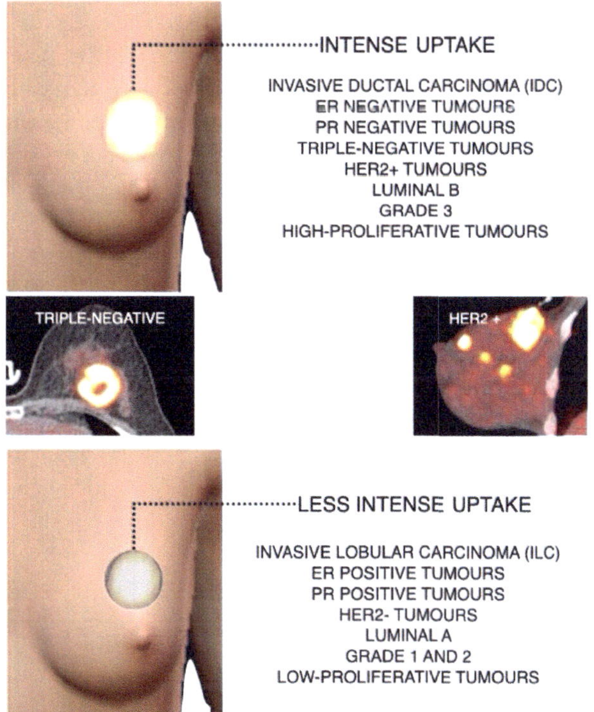

1.13 ¹⁸F-FDG PET/CT to Assess Metastatic Disease in Breast Cancer

^{18}F-FDG PET/CT has high diagnostic accuracy for the evaluation of regional and distant metastases in patients with inflammatory and locally advanced breast cancer. It can detect distant metastases in >20% of patients with locally advanced breast cancer corresponding to AJCC stages IIIC, IIIB and IIIA (except for T3N1 tumours).

Therapeutic impact of changing management from curative to palliative is 1–8% in early breast cancer, 7–13% in locally advanced breast cancer and up to 52% in inflammatory breast cancer but has no impact on cN0 early breast cancer.

^{18}F-FDG PET/CT can distinguish involved lymph nodes located at axillary Berg level III (infraclavicular area, supero-medial to the pectoralis minor muscle) from those located in the lower axillary levels I and II. However, compared to SN biopsy ^{18}F-FDG PET/CT has poorer sensitivity for axillary nodal metastases. Nevertheless, the modality can assess regional node disease outside the axilla (supraclavicular area and internal mammary chain) which is less commonly identified by SN evaluation. When ^{18}F-FDG PET/CT is used in conjunction with ultrasonography for the assessment of nodal disease the accuracy improves to more than 90%.

With the exception of brain metastases ^{18}F-FDG PET/CT is very effective in detecting occult distant metastases. In skeleton ^{18}F-FDG PET/CT is more sensitive and specific than bone scan and contrast-enhancement CT to detect lytic or mixed bone metastases, or bone marrow involvement. By contrast in osteoblastic metastases FDG uptake is more variable and is often less sensitive than bone scintigraphy.

^{18}F-FDG PET/CT is quite effective in detecting distal nodal disease as well as pleural, hepatic, splenic, adrenal, and pelvic metastases. By contrast, it is less sensitive than thorax CT which could be explained by the partial volume effect and respiratory motion that affect ^{18}F-FDG PET/CT.

The detection of metastases by ^{18}F-FDG PET/CT differs according to the characteristics of the primary tumour. For distant lymph node metastases FDG uptake is higher for grade-3, in triple negative, and HER2+ tumours. Although the rate of distant metastases is not necessarily related to tumour grade or breast cancer subtype the distribution of metastases varies according to breast cancer subtype: for instance, triple negative and HER2+ tumours show more extra-skeletal metastases than OR+/HER2- tumours. A relative higher rate of clinically unsuspected stage IV disease has been found in younger patients (>40 years) at lower TNM stages, suggesting that clinical TNM staging may not be the only relevant factor on which decision to perform a staging ^{18}F-FDG PET/CT should be based.

With respect to the recently introduced ^{18}F-FDG PET/MRI this modality has demonstrated to achieve similar diagnostic performance in comparison to ^{18}F-FDG PET/CT with no statistically significant differences in nodal staging and even higher accuracy in overall distant staging of metastases. The main reason for the higher sensitivity of PET/MRI comes from non-FDG avid lesions such as permeative osseous metastases and subcentimeter hepatic metastases that are visible on MRI but not on CT.

PET/CT has a high positive predictive value to stage the axilla in N$^+$ patients and therefore to stratify risk by estimating tumour load based on the number of ^{18}F-FDG avid axillary lymph nodes. Besides cN1 (1–3 positive lymph nodes), who are considered low-risk, cN2 (4 or more positive lymph nodes) are considered high-risk needing additional radiotherapy [9, 40–43].

^{18}F-FDG PET/CT AND METASTATIC DISEASE

N+ REGIONAL METASTASES

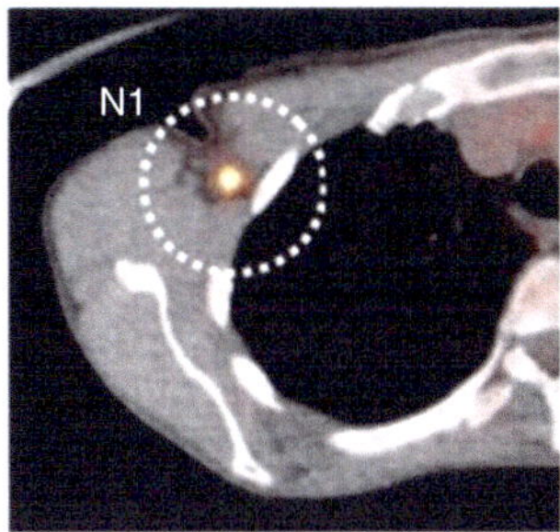

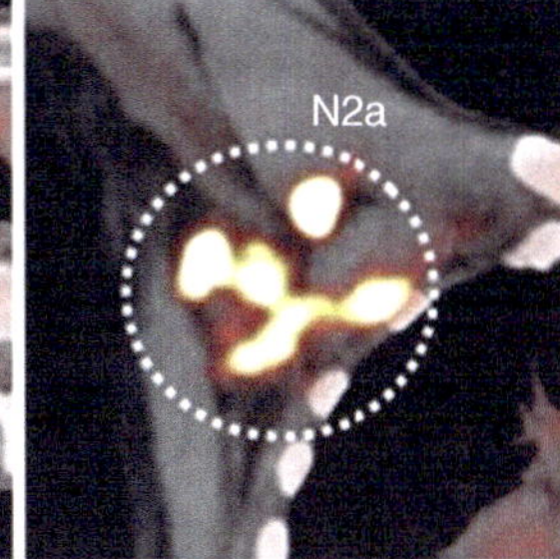

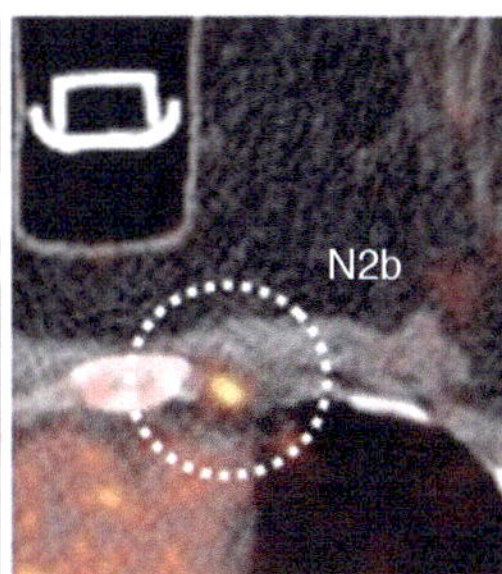

AXILLARY LYMPH NODE METASTASES

INTERNAL MAMMARY

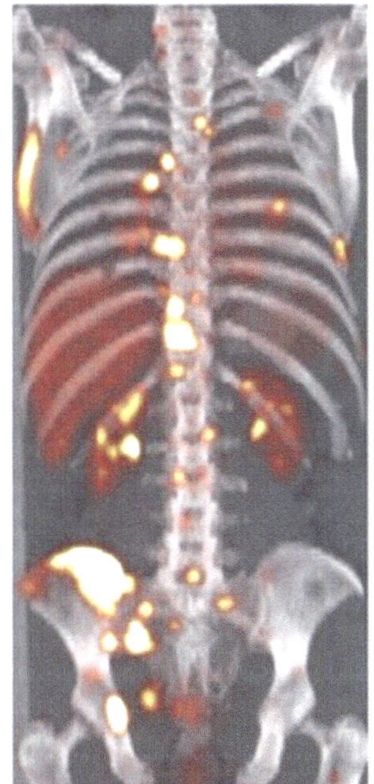

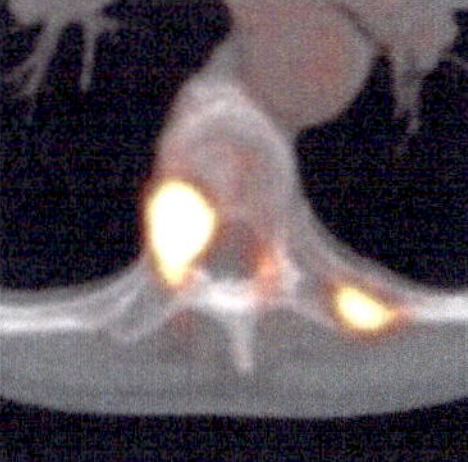

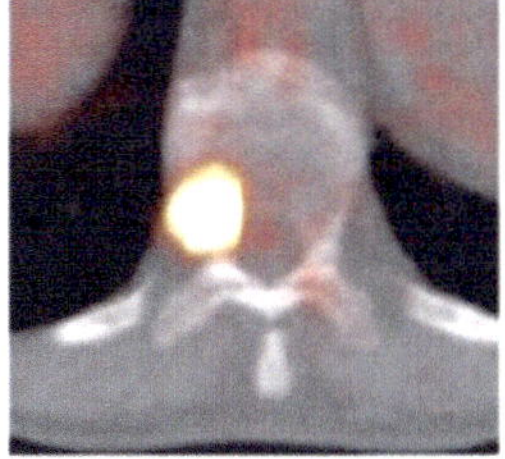

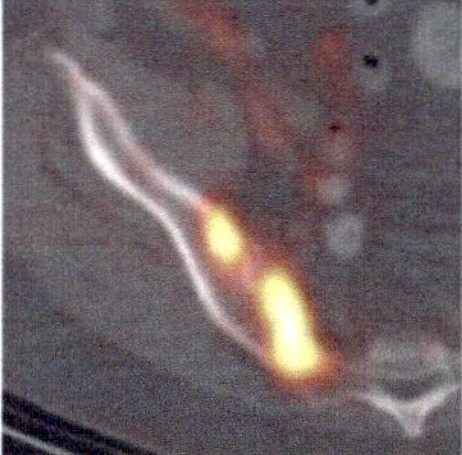

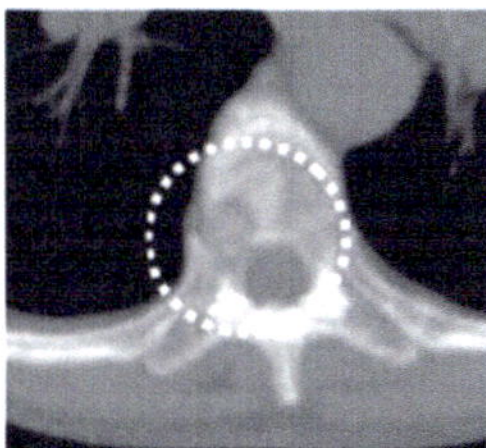

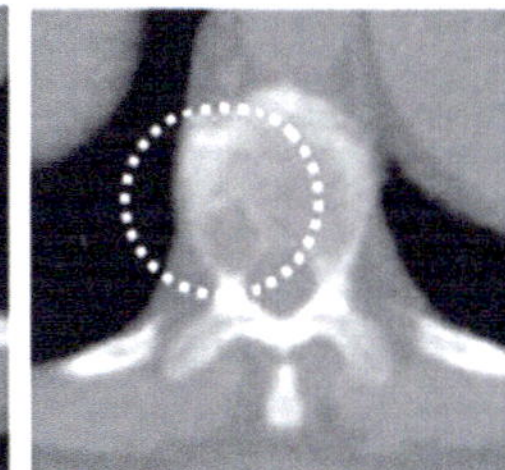

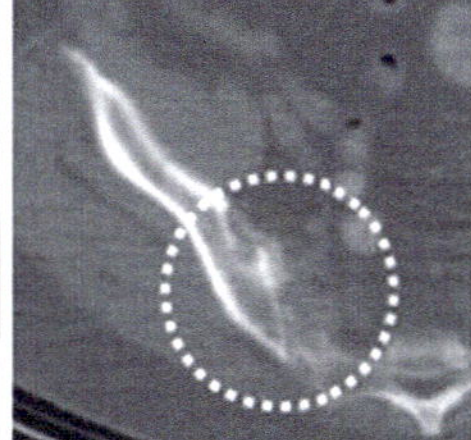

^{18}F-FDG AVID LYTIC BONE METASTASES

M1 DISTANT METASTASES

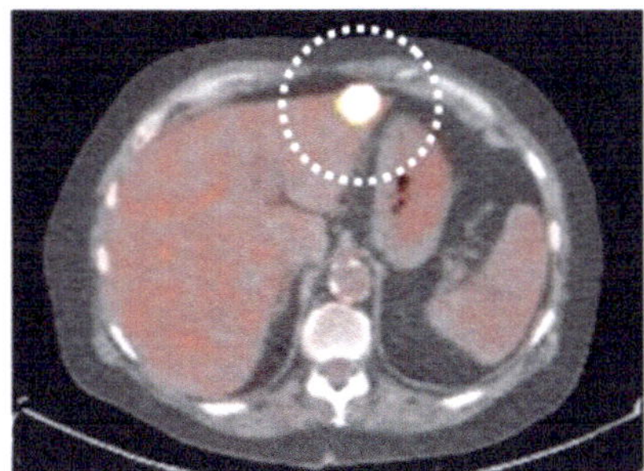

^{18}F-FDG AVID LIVER METASTASIS

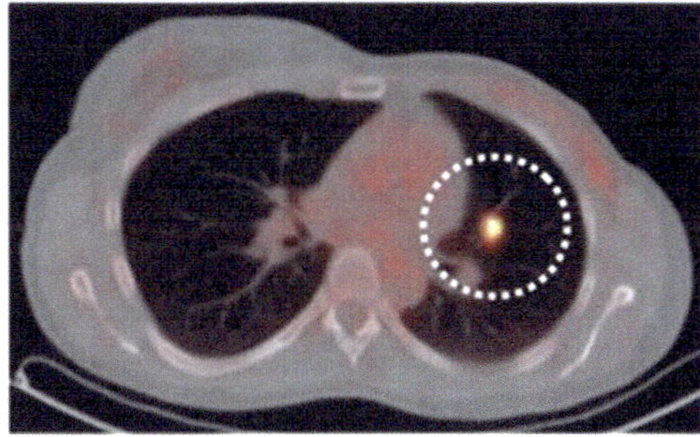

^{18}F-FDG AVID LUNG METASTATSIS

1.14 Methodological Aspects of ^{18}F-FDG PET/CT

Guidelines for patient preparation include no exercise the day before examination to prevent muscular uptake, no consumption of foods or liquids other than unflavoured water for at last 6 hours before ^{18}F-FDG administration, patient needs to be kept warm to prevent ^{18}F-FDG uptake in brown fat, blood glucose needs to be lower than 10 mmol/l to prevent altered tracer biodistribution.

Usually, patients receive a single intravenous ^{18}F-FDG dose of 180–240 MBq depending on their body mass index and (sensitivity of the) PET/CT system. ^{18}F-FDG needs to be administered with the patient lying comfortably to minimize muscular uptake. Injection in the upper extremity contralateral to the primary breast malignancy to prevent artefacts like lymph node uptake in the ipsilateral axilla. After tracer administration a resting period of approximately 60 minutes is necessary.

Whole body PET/CT acquisition, usually from crown to mid-thigh, with the patient in supine position is the standard for the evaluation of distal metastases in breast cancer.

Complementary PET/CT of the thorax with the patient in prone position using a mock-up coil is recommended for assessment of locoregional staging. This dedicated hanging breast imaging performs better than supine in evaluating the number of involved lymph nodes and improves visualization of primary tumour extension and multifocality.

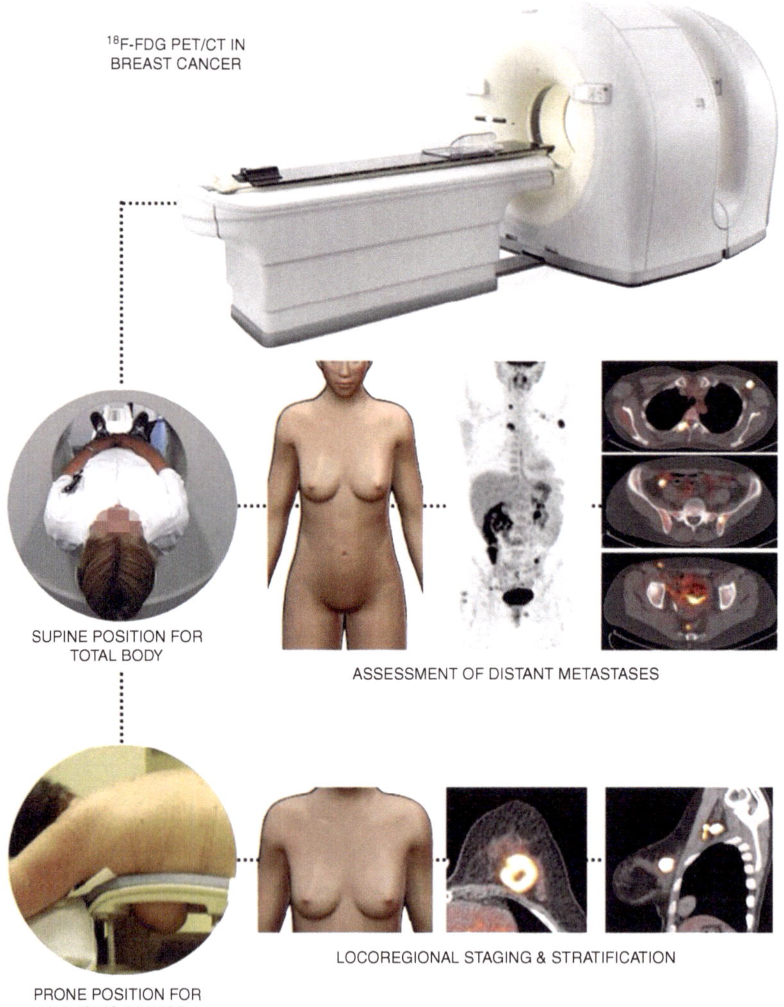

Image reading includes a description of the number of ^{18}F-FDG lesions in the affected and contralateral breast, ipsilateral axilla, extra-axillary and at distance. Localization needs to accurately be effectuated in order to facilitate correlation with MRI and/of diagnostic CT. Concerning primary tumours aspects such as location related to breast quadrant and/or clock-face need to be reported as well as lesion depth in relation to nipple. In analogy with the lexicon used for dedicated breast PET and MBI a four-step score (0: no uptake, 1: slight uptake, 2: moderate uptake, 3: very intense uptake) in relation to background activity (breast parenchyma uptake) may be useful to characterize breast lesions. In the axilla, the number of ^{18}F-FDG avid lymph nodes is important in order to stratify risk (cN1 with1–3 positive lymph nodes is considered low-risk, cN2 with 4 or more positive lymph nodes is considered high risk). In addition, suspected extra-axillary lesions should be described including their precise localization and anatomical substrate. Assessment of SUVmax and other parameters of index lesions is recommended to characterize malignancy and to enable therapy response [41, 44, 45].

1.15 Breast Cancer Molecular Imaging with Non-^{18}F-FDG PET Tracers

Evaluation of HER2 expression. In biopsies, there are two different possibilities to evaluate HER2 status: immunohistochemistry (IHC) to detect HER2 protein overexpression and fluorescence in situ hybridization (FISH) to detect HER2 gene amplification. However, both IHC and FISH may not translate the status of HER2 expression of the whole tumour and/or metastases. In this respect, whole body molecular imaging to characterize HER2 distribution is a promising alternative. Attempts to accomplish this objective have led to the radiolabelling of humanized monoclonal antibodies such as ^{64}Cu-DOTA-trastuzumab, ^{89}Zr-trastuzumab and ^{89}Zr-pertuzumab to target HER2 which have the potential to detect unsuspected HER2-positive foci contributing to appropriate HER2-targeted therapy. Another route for HER2 assessment is the use of a HER2-binding affibody molecule which has resulted in the development of ^{68}Ga-ABY-025.

Oestrogen receptor (OR) imaging. The use of oestrogen derivatives labelled with PET tracers may be of crucial importance to assess the intra-tumour heterogeneity of OR expression which is responsible for the variable biopsy results in some breast carcinomas as well as to assess the heterogeneity of OR expression in metastatic breast cancer. In this field ^{18}F-fluoroestradiol (^{18}F-FES) combines high sensitivity and specificity to measure the OR status in breast cancer (metastases) and its uptake may guide therapy selection and endocrine treatment response. In addition, it may be useful in diagnostic dilemmas when conventional imaging techniques including ^{18}F-FDG PET/CT do not suffice, for example in low-grade ILC. The alternative PET tracer 4-Fluoro-11β-methoxy-16α-18F-fluoroestradiol (^{18}F-4FMFES) shows a tumour uptake quite similar to ^{18}F-FES but with an improved target-to-non-target ratio leading to a greater sensitivity for breast cancers overexpressing OR.

Progesterone receptor (PR) imaging. PR expression has a strong prognostic value since metastatic breast cancer positive for both OR and PR shows more response to hormone therapy in comparison to cancer with OR positivity but lacks PR expression. ^{18}F-FFNP (^{18}F-fluoro-16α,17α-[(R)-(1′-α-furymethylidene)dyoxy]-19-norpregn-4=ene-3,30-dione) can measure the PR expression by means of PET even when OR is blocked, which is advantageous in comparison to ^{18}F-FES.

Anti-1-amino-3-^{18}F-fluorocyclobutane-1-carboxylic acid (^{18}F-FACBC or ^{18}F-fluciclovine) is a synthetic amino acid analogue, which may be useful in staging ILC, since its uptake in this breast cancer type tends to be higher than uptake of ^{18}F-FDG.

Recently, the fibroblast activation protein inhibitor (FAPI) labelled with^{68}Ga (^{68}Ga-FAPI-04) has been found to be more sensitive than ^{18}F-FDG in detecting primary breast lesions as well as distant metastases [46–48].

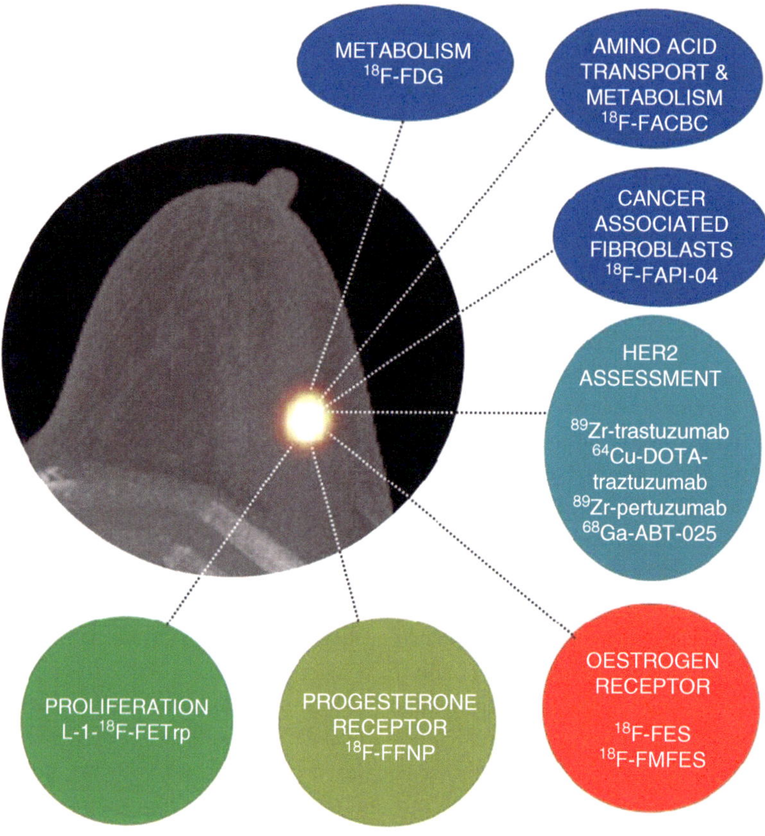
METABOLISM
^{18}F-FDG
AMINO ACID TRANSPORT & METABOLISM
^{18}F-FACBC
CANCER ASSOCIATED FIBROBLASTS
^{18}F-FAPI-04
HER2 ASSESSMENT
^{89}Zr-trastuzumab
^{64}Cu-DOTA-traztuzumab
^{89}Zr-pertuzumab
^{68}Ga-ABT-025
PROLIFERATION
L-1-^{18}F-FETrp
PROGESTERONE RECEPTOR
^{18}F-FFNP
OESTROGEN RECEPTOR
^{18}F-FES
^{18}F-FMFES
PER-TRACERS IN BREAST CANCER

1.16 Dedicated Breast PET

Although refinement of PET/CT acquisition with a complementary study in prone position may resolve various limitations related to detection and characterization of primary breast lesions, both limited spatial resolution and the need for specific acquisition parameters may limit the routine application of PET/CT scanners in the diagnosis of primary breast cancer, especially in small-sized lesions.

The limitations related to conventional PET/CT scanners have led to the development of breast-specific PET systems that recognize two types: systems based on compression of the breast and devices using hanging breast imaging.

Breast compression devices were the first to be introduced and are known as positron emission mammography (PEM) in the literature. PEM uses two planar detectors placed on either side of the breast with the patient positioned in a similar manner as in mammography. The most popular of these devices is the PEM Flex Solo II scanner from Naviscan, which consists of two opposing lutetium-yttrium oxyorthosilicate (LYSO) crystal-based PET detectors that move linearly within compression paddles placed on either side of a gently stabilized breast. Patients are seated upright and positioned in either craniocaudal or mediolateral oblique positions.

PEM appears to be more sensitive than PET/CT using ^{18}F-FDG varying from 73% (vs. 60%) for T1a or T1b, 95% (vs. 84%) for T1c and 100% (vs. 95%) for T2 tumours. Based on a meta-analysis pooled sensitivity and specificity scored 85% and 79%, respectively. Missed cancers were usually small or outside the field of view.

Out of the hanging breast systems MAMMI (MAMography with Molecular Imaging) PET is one of the most used devices. It is a true tomographic ring scanner using LYSO-based PET detectors. Breasts are separately imaged with the patient in prone position. No compression is applied.

MAMMI PET has a higher sensitivity than PET/CT in detecting primary breast cancer lesions except for tumours located outside the scanning range of the device in areas close to the pectoral muscle. To solve this limitation the use of a larger circular aperture to position the hanging breast in the imaging table of the device has been recommended.

MAMMI PET is a better device than PET/CT to evaluate the heterogeneity of tumour ^{18}F-FDG uptake in large lesions. With respect to tumour uptake a four-step score in relation to background activity (breast parenchyma uptake) helps to characterize breast lesions: 0: no uptake, 1: slight uptake, 2: moderate uptake, 3: very intense uptake. This score can be added to the lexicon proposed for breast lesions incorporating location (breast quadrant and/or clock-face), lesion depth (related to nipple) and likelihood of malignancy (complementing BI-RADS scale).

A ring-type dedicated breast PET (similar to MAMMI) has been found to have a higher sensitivity than PET/CT for subcentimeter tumours (81.9% vs. 52.4%) in a large cohort of patients. With the exception of lobular carcinoma in situ dedicated breast PET appears to be superior for all histologic types that show low sensitivity of detection on PET/CT [49–52].

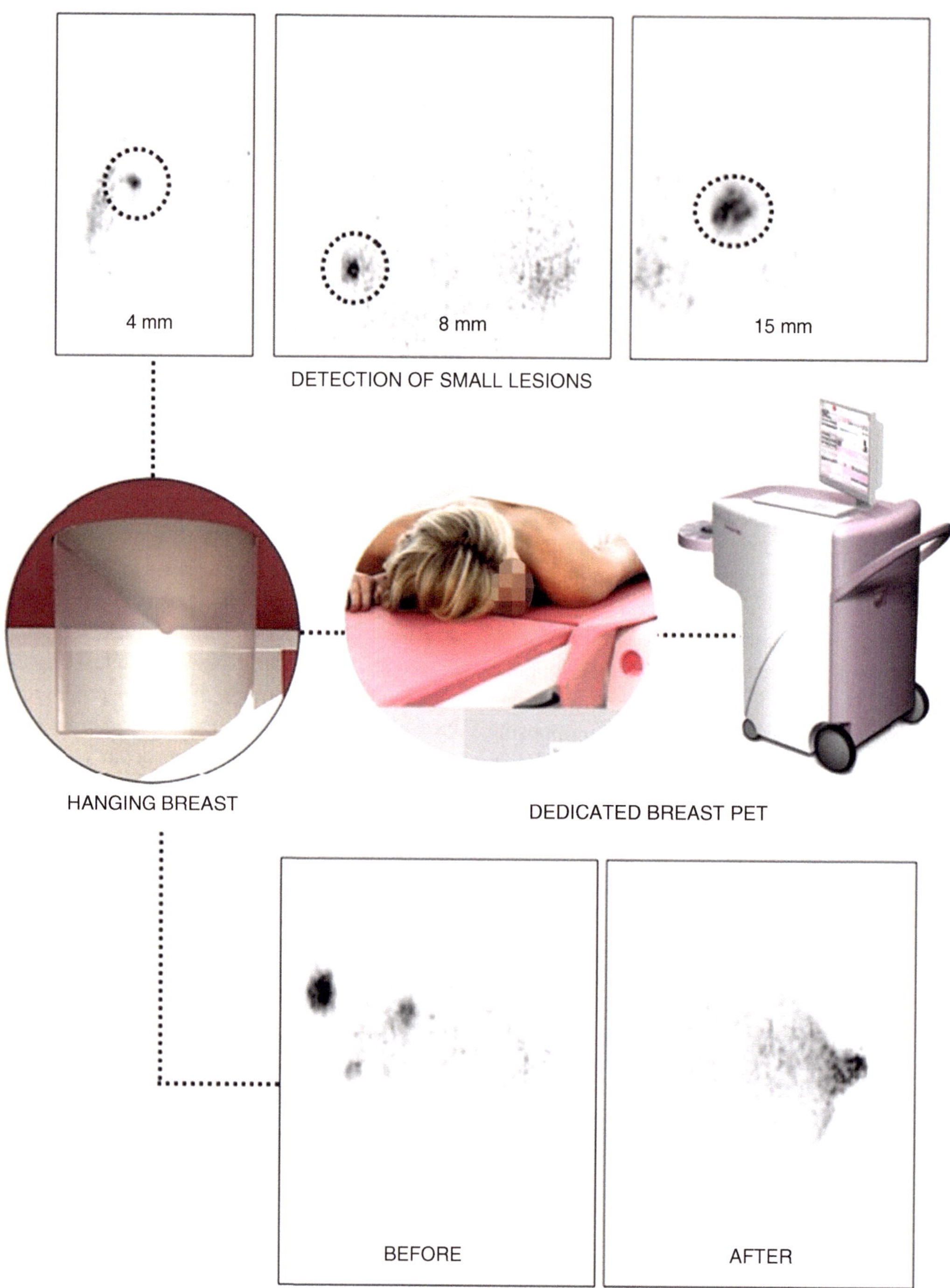
4 mm
8 mm
15 mm
DETECTION OF SMALL LESIONS
HANGING BREAST
DEDICATED BREAST PET
BEFORE
AFTER
ASSESSMENT OF THERAPY RESPONSE

1.17 Molecular Breast Imaging with ^{99m}Tc-sestamibi for Lesion Detection and Biopsy

Different from mammography and ultrasound Molecular Breast Imaging (MBI) is a physiologic approach to breast cancer detection.

MBI, also called breast-specific gamma imaging (BSGI), is able to detect occult additional foci in 9% of newly diagnosed breast cancer, 97% of invasive breast cancer and 91% of ductal carcinoma in situ.

MBI/BSGI detects occult cancer in up to 16.5 per 1000 women, is increasingly being used in assessing response to neoadjuvant chemotherapy, and, due to its high sensitivity (95%), is of complementary value for breast cancer screening in patients with dense breast.

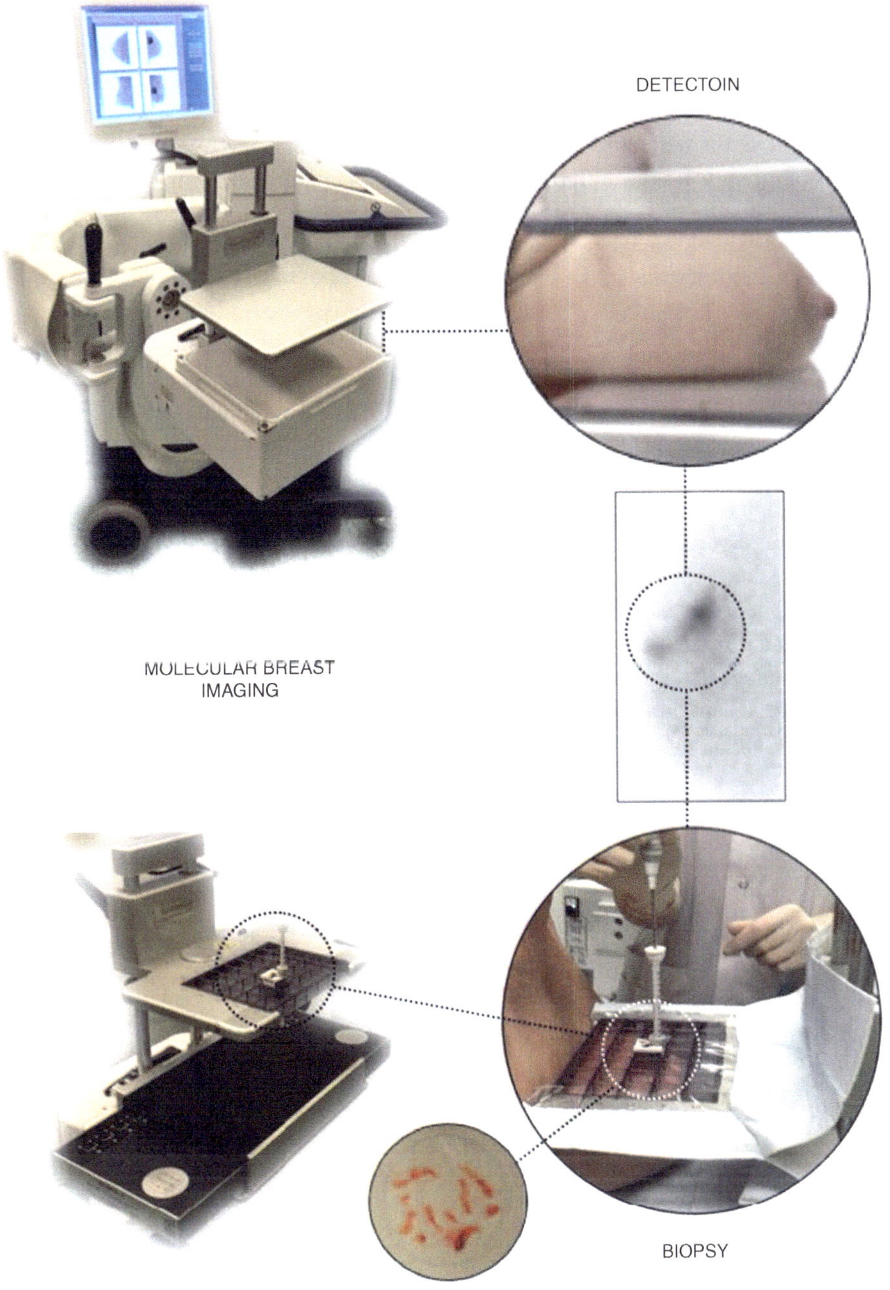

Some other clinical indications are the evaluation of: local breast cancer recurrence, extent of disease in recently detected breast malignancy, BI-RADS 3 lesions, enhancing areas seen on MRI, palpable abnormalities not demonstrated on mammography or ultrasound, multiple masses demonstrated on breast imaging, occult breast cancer in cases of axillary lymph node metastases with unknown primary, suspected malignancy in patients with technically difficult mammography (implants, free silicone or paraffin injections, radiodense breasts) or MRI (implanted pacemakers or pumps, ferromagnetic surgical implants, claustrophobia, renal disease etc.).

In patients with undetermined mammographic findings (BI-RADS 0) MBI appears to change management in more than 90% of the cases versus 40% for ultrasound.

Although MBI reliably images subcentimeter cancers some posterior lesions in the breast may be located out of the field of view which may reduce their sensitivity.

MBI is performed 5–10 min after intravenous injection of ^{99m}Tc-sestamibi in the contralateral arm when the affected breast is known in order to avoid lymph node uptake from eventual extravasation. The patient is seated during the entire study with the breast gently compressed between the gamma detector and a compression plate when a one-head device is used, or between both detectors with a dual-headed camera and bilateral conventional craniocaudal and mediolateral oblique views are acquired allowing direct comparison with mammography.

Visual lesion uptake can be characterized in relation to subcutaneous fat intensity as photopenic (less intense), mild (equal or slightly greater), moderate (greater than mild but less than twice as intense as subcutaneous fat) and marked (at least twice the intensity of subcutaneous fat).

In addition to type and intensity of uptake, the location and size of focal lesions are reported in a similar manner as outlined in mammography for BI-RADS providing information about breast quadrant or clock-face and distance to the nipple.

Based on lesion characteristics a BI-RADS model tailored for MBI assessment has been proposed: 0—incomplete (needs additional imaging); 1—negative (routine follow-up); 2—benign (routine follow-up); 3—very low likelihood of malignancy (follow-up in 6 months if targeted diagnostic mammogram and ultrasound are negative); 4—suspicious (consider biopsy); 5—highly suggestive of malignancy (take appropriate action); 6—known malignancy (take appropriate action).

MBI-guided breast lesion biopsy is performed using a sliding slant-hole collimator in order to calculate lesion depth. Starting 5 min after ^{99m}Tc-sestamibi injection the procedure time is approximately 75 min including stereotactic images, X/Y/Z lesion localization, needle placement and verification as well as biopsy. MBI biopsy is principally indicated in patients with lesions not depicted on mammography or ultrasound but suspicious on MBI (assessment criteria 4–5) [50, 53–57].

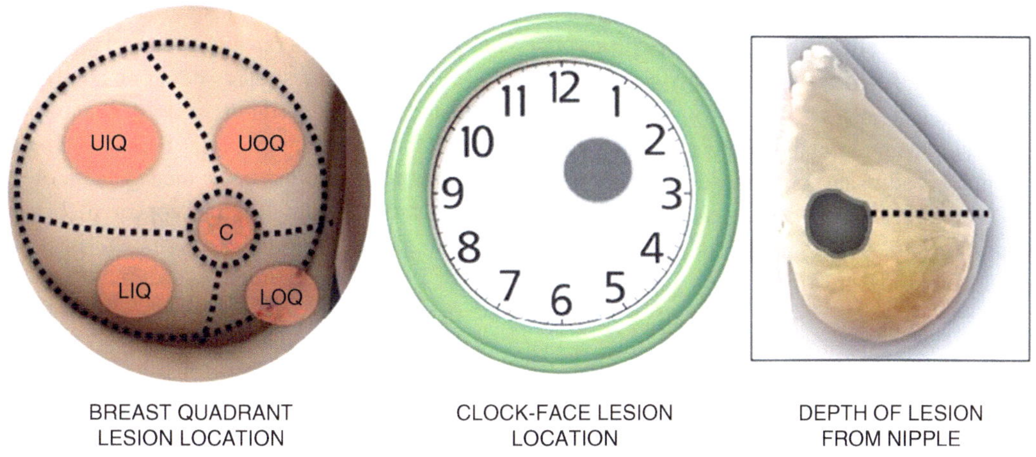

LEXICON FOR STANDARDISED INTERPRETATION OF MOLECULAR BREAST IMAGING & DEDICATED PET

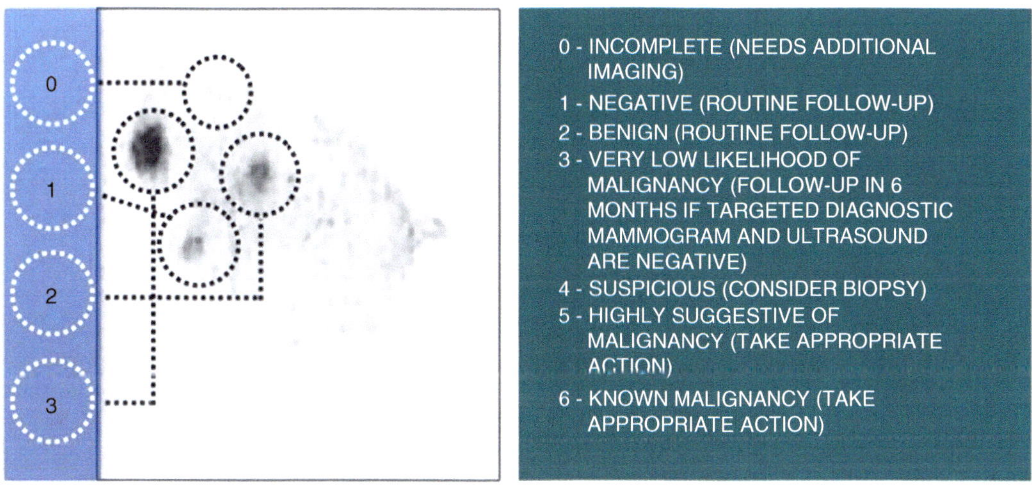

1.18 New Interventional Nuclear Medicine-Based Strategies for Axillary Management

In patients with resectable early-stage breast carcinoma neoadjuvant systemic treatment (NST) has become a standard of care and the pattern of response is an essential aspect to tailor systemic and locoregional treatment. This approach may lead to an escalating treatment in non-responders and de-escalating therapy in responders.

In this context, a strategy based on combining validated nuclear medicine procedures may be useful for the management of the axilla. An example may be found in the management of the node-positive axilla. Patients appear to benefit from a specific algorithm combining [^{18}F]FDG PET/CT and a radioguided procedure.

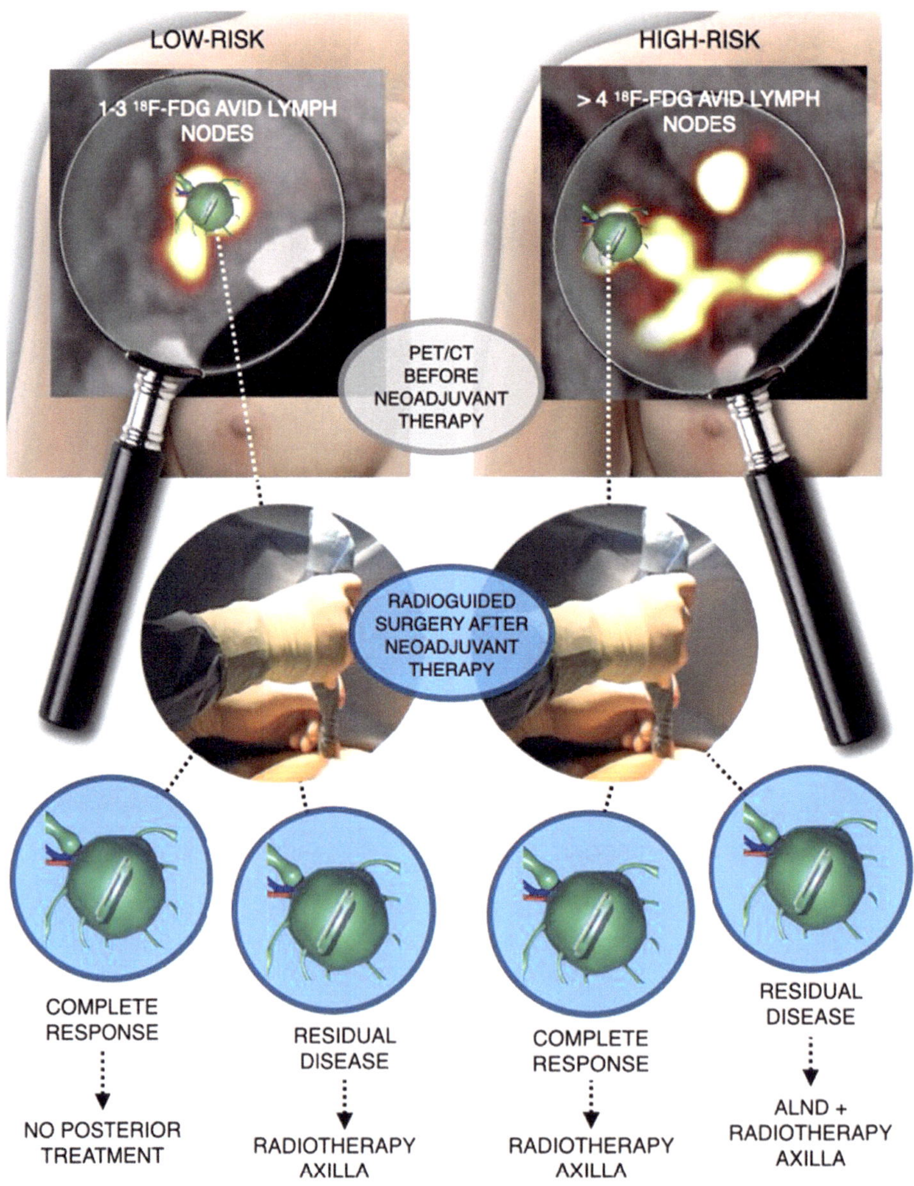

[18F]FDG has a high positive predictive value to stage and stratify the axilla prior to NST. In addition, the MARI technique for marking involved axillary lymph nodes with radioactive iodine seeds has an acceptable false-negative rate in predicting complete response or residual axillary disease posterior to NST.

The application of this strategy enables risk stratification and tailoring of management of the axilla. In patients with 1–3 [18F]FDG avid lymph nodes and MARI complete response no subsequent treatment is proposed whereas in patients with residual disease radiotherapy of the axilla is applied. On the other hand, patients with more than 4 [18F] FDG avid lymph nodes and MARI associated with complete response are candidates for radiotherapy of the axilla whereas for patients with MARI-associated residual disease both axillary lymph node dissection and radiotherapy are proposed.

The application of this algorithm resulted in an 82% reduction in axillary lymph node dissection with a low recurrence rate on follow-up. The additional incorporation of SN biopsy to MARI procedure contributes to further reducing the false-negative rates when the approach is combined [58–61].

References

1. American Cancer Society. Breast cancer facts & figures 2019-2020. Atlanta: American Cancer Society, Inc; 2019.
2. Ferlay J, Colombet M, Soerjomataram I, et al. Cancer incidence and mortality patterns in Europe: estimates for 40 countries and 25 major cancers in 2018. Eur J Cancer. 2018;103:356–87.
3. Sung H, Ferlay J, Siegel RL, et al. Global cancer statistics 2020: GLOBOSCAN estimates of incidence and mortality worldwide for 36 cancer in 185 countries. CA Cancer J Clin. 2021;0:1–41. https://doi.org/10.3322/caac.21660.
4. Giuliano AE, Connolly JL, Edge SB, et al. Breast cancer – major changes in the American joint committee on cancer eighth edition cancer staging manual. CA Cancer J Clin. 2017;67:290–303.
5. Johnson KS, Conant EF, Scott SM. Molecular subtypes of breast cancer: a review for breast radiologists. J Breast Imaging. 2021;3:12–24.
6. Amin MB, Greene FL, Byrd DR, et al., editors. AJCC cancer staging manual. 8th ed. Springer International Publishing; 2017.
7. Brierley JD, Gospodarowicz MK, Wittekind C, editors. TNM classification of malignant tumours. 8th ed. Hoboken: Wiley Blackwell; 2017.
8. Cardoso F, Kyriakides S, Ohno S, et al. Early breast cancer: ESMO clinical practice guidelines for diagnosis, treatment and follow-up. Ann Oncol. 2019;30:1194–220.
9. Chung HL, Le-Petross HT, Leung JWT. Imaging updates to breast cancer lymph node management. Radiographics. 2021;41:1283–99.
10. Kalli S, Semine A, Cohen S, et al. American Joint Committee on cancer's staging system for breast cancer, eighth edition: what the radiologist needs to know. Radiographics. 2018;38:1921–33.
11. Berg JW. The significance of axillary node levels in the study of breast carcinoma. Cancer. 1955;8:776–8.
12. Clough KB, Nasr R, Nos C, Vieira C, Inguenault C, Pulet B. New anatomical classification of the axilla with implications for sentinel node biopsy. Br J Surg. 2010;97:1659–65.
13. Uren RF, Howman-Giles R, Chung DKV, Spillane AJ, Noushi F, Gillet D, Gluch L, Mak C, West R, Briody J, Carmalt H. SPECT/CT scans allow precise anatomical location of sentinel lymph nodes in breast cancer and redefine lymphatic drainage from the breast to the axilla. Breast. 2012;21:480–6.
14. James TA, Palis B, McCabe R, Pardo JA, Alapati A, Ukandu O, Serres SK, Zhang J, Mele A, Facktor M, Shulman LN. Evaluating the role of sentinel lymph node biopsy in patients with DCIS treated with breast conserving surgery. Am J Surg. 2020;220:654–9.
15. Lyman GH, Somerfield MR, Bosserman LD, Perkins CL, Weaver DL, Giuliano AE. Sentinel lymph node biopsy for patients with early-stage breast cancer: American Society of Clinical Oncology clinical practice guide update. J Clin Oncol. 2017;35:561–4.
16. Niebling MG, Pleijhuis RG, Bastiaannet E, Brouwers AH, van Dam GM, Hoekstra HJ. A systematic review and meta-analyses of sentinel lymph node identification in breast cancer and melanoma, a plea for tracer imaging. Eur J Surg. 2016;42:466–73.
17. Tanis PJ, Nieweg OE, Valdés Olmos RA, Rutgers EJT, Kroon BBR. History of sentinel node and validation of the technique. Breast Cancer Res. 2001;3:109–12.
18. Van Loevezijn AA, Bartels SAL, van Duijnhoven FH, Heemsbergen WD, Bosma SJ, Elkhuizen PHM, Donswijk ML, Rutgers EJT, Oldenburg HSA, Vrancken Peeters MTFD, van der Ploeg IMC. Internal mammary chain sentinel nodes in early-stage breast cancer patients: toward selective removal. Ann Surg Oncol. 2019;26:945–53.
19. Borrelli P, Donswijk ML, Stokkel MP, Teixeira SC, van Tinteren, Rutgers EJT, Valdés Olmos RA. Contribution of SPECT/CT for sentinel node localization in patients with ipsilateral breast cancer relapse. Eur J Nucl Med Mol Imaging. 2017;44:630–7.
20. Giammarile F, Alazraki N, Aarsvold JN, Audisio RA, Glass E, Grant SF, Kunikowska J, Leidenius M, Moncayo VM, Uren RF, Oyen WJG, Valdés Olmos RA, Vidal SS. The EANM and SNMMI practice

guideline for lymphoscintigraphy and sentinel node localization in breast cancer. Eur J Nucl Med Mol Imaging. 2013;40:1932–47.
21. Jimenez-Hefferman A, Ellman A, Sado H, Huíc D, Bal C, Parameswaran R, Giammarile F, Pruzzo R, Kostadinova I, Vorster M, Almeida P, Santiago J, Gambhir S, Sergieva S, Calderon A, Oh Young G, Valdes-Olmos R, Zaknun J, Magboo VP, Pascual TNB. Results of a prospective multicenter International Atomic Energy Agency sentinel node trial on the value of SPECT/CT over planar imaging in various malignancies. J Nucl Med. 2015;56:1338–44.
22. Chahid Y, Qiu X, van de Garde EMW, Verberne HJ, Booij J. Risk factors for nonvisualization of the sentinel lymph node on lymphoscintigraphy in breast cancer patients. EJNMI Res. 2021;11:54.
23. Estourgie SH, Nieweg OE, Valdés Olmos RA, Rutgers EJT, Kroon BBR. Lymphatic drainage patterns from the breast. Ann Surg. 2004;239:232–7.
24. Freebody J, Fernando S, Rossleigh MA. Triple-site radiotracer application in breast lymphoscitigraphy and sentinel node discordance. World J Nucl Med. 2019;18:127–31.
25. Pereira Arias-Bouda LM, Vidal-Sicart S, Valdés Olmos RA. Preoperative and intraoperative lymphatic mapping for radioguided sentinel lymph node biopsy in breast cancer. In: Mariani G, Vidal-Sicart S, Valdés Olmos RA, editors. Atlas of lymphoscintigraphy and sentinel node mapping. Milan: Springer; 2020. p. 185–217.
26. Tanis PJ, Valdés Olmos RA, Muller SH, Nieweg OE. Lymphatic mapping in patients with breast carcinoma: reproducibility of lymphoscintigraphc results. Radiology. 2003;228:546–51.
27. Bartoli F, Bisogni G, Vitali S, Cataldi AG, Del Guerra A, Mariani G, Erba PA. Methodological aspects of lymphatic mapping: radiopharmaceuticals, multimodal lymphatic mapping, agents, instrumentations. In: Mariani G, Vidal-Sicart S, Valdés Olmos RA, editors. Atlas of lymphoscintigraphy and sentinel node mapping. Milan: Springer; 2020. p. 21–51.
28. Orsini F, Guidoccio F, Vidal-Sicart S, Valdés Olmos RA, Mariani G. General concepts on radioguided sentinel lymph node biopsy: preoperative imaging, intraoperative gamma probe guidance, intraoperative imaging, multimodality imaging. In: Mariani G, Vidal-Sicart S, Valdés Olmos RA, editors. Atlas of lymphoscintigraphy and sentinel node mapping. Milan: Springer; 2020. p. 151–69.
29. Paganelli G, De Cicco C, Gatti G, Luini A. Radioguided occult lesion localization in the breast. In: Mariani G, Giuliano AE, Strauss HW, editors. Radioguided surgery – a comprehensive team approach. New York: Springer; 2008. p. 81–91.
30. van Rijk MC, Tanis PJ, Nieweg OE, Loo CE, Valdés Olmos RA, Oldenburg HS, Rutgers EJ, Hoefnagel CA, Kroon BB. Sentinel node biopsy and concomitant probe-guided tumor excision of nonpalpable breast cancer. Ann Surg Oncol. 2007;14:627–32.
31. Donker M, Drukker CA, Valdés Olmos RA, Rutgers EJ, Loo CE, Sonke GS, et al. Guiding breast-conserving surgery in patients after neoadjuvant systemic therapy for breast cancer: a comparison of radioactive seed localization with the ROLL technique. Ann Surg Oncol. 2013;20:2569–75.
32. Gray RJ, Salud C, Nguyen K, Dauway E, Friedland J, Berman C, Peltz E, et al. Randomized prospective evaluation of a novel technique for biopsy or lumpectomy of nonpalpable breast lesions: radioactive seed versus wire localization. Ann Surg Oncol. 2001;8:711–5.
33. Niinikoski L, Hukkinen K, Leidenius MHK, Vaara P, Voynov A, Heikkilä P, et al. Resection margins and local recurrences of impalpable breast cancer: comparison between radioguided occult lesion localization (ROLL) and radioactive seed localization (RSL). Breast. 2019;47:93–101.
34. Wright CM, Moorin RE, Saunders C, Marinovich ML, Taylor DB, Bourke AG, et al. Cost-effectiveness of radioguided occult lesion localization using 125I seeds versus hookwire localization before breast-conserving surgery for non-palpable breast cancer. Br J Surg. 2021;108:843–50.
35. Banys-Paluchowski M, Gasparri ML, de Boniface J, Gentilini O, Stickeler E, Hartmann S, et al. Surgical management of the axilla in clinically node-positive breast cancer patients converting to clinical node negativity through neoadjuvant chemotherapy: current status, knowledge gaps, and rationale for the EUBREAST-03 AXSANA study. Cancers. 2021;13:1565.
36. Donker M, Straver ME, Wesseling J, Loo CE, Schot M, Drukker CA, et al. Marking axillary lymph nodes with radioactive iodine seeds for axillary staging after neoadjuvant systemic treatment in breast cancer patients: the MARI procedure. Ann Surg. 2015;261:378–82.
37. Hassing CMS, Tvedskov TF, Kroman N, Klausen TL, Drejøe JB, Tvedskov JF, et al. Radioactive seed localization of non-palpable lymph nodes – a feasibility study. Eur J Surg Oncol. 2018;44:725–30.
38. Straver ME, Loo CE, Alderliesten T, Rutgers EJT, Vrancken Peeters MTFD. Marking the axilla with radioactive iodine seeds (MARI procedure) may reduce the need for axillary dissection after neoadjuvant chemotherapy for breast cancer. Br J Surg. 2010;97:1226–31.
39. Aroztegui AP, García Vicente AM, Alvarez Ruiz S, Delgado Bolton RC, Orcajo Rincón J, García Garzon JR, et al. 18F-FDG PET/CT in breast cancer: evidence-based recommendations in initial staging. Tumor Biol. 2017:1–23.
40. Groheux D, Hindle E. Breast cancer: initial workup and staging with FDG PET/CT. Clin Trans Imaging. 2021;9:221–31.
41. Ulaner GA. PET/CT for patients with breast cancer: where is the clinical impact? Am J Roentgenol. 2019;213:254–65.

42. de Mooij CM, Sunen I, Mitea C, Lalji UC, Vanwestswinkel S, Smidt ML, et al. Diagnostic performance of PET/computed tomography versus PET/MRI and diffusion-weighted imaging in the N- and M-staging of breast cancer patients. Nucl Med Commun. 2020;41:995–1004.
43. Teixeira SC, Koolen BB, Elkhuizen PHM, Vrancken Peeters MJTFD, Stokkel MPM, Rodenhuis S, et al. PET/CT with ^{18}F-FDG predicts short-term outcome in stage II/III breast cancer patients upstaged to N2/3 nodal disease. Eur J Surg Oncol. 2017;43:625–35.
44. Abramson RG, Lambert KF, Jones-Jackson LB, Arlinghaus LR, Williams J, Abramson VG, et al. Prone versus supine breast FDG-PET/CT for assessing locoregional disease distribution in locally advanced breast cancer. Acad Radiol. 2015;22:853–9.
45. Teixeira SC, Koolen BB, Vogel WV, Wesseling J, Stokkel MP, Vrancken Peeters MJTFD, et al. Additional prone 18F-FDG PET/CT acquisition to improve the visualization of the primary tumor and regional lymph node metastases in stage II/III breast cancer. Clin Nucl Med. 2016a;41:e181–6.
46. Abrantes AM, Pires AS, Monteiro L, Teixo R, Neves AR, Tavares NT, et al. Tumour functional imaging by PET. Biochim Biophys Acta Mol basis Dis. 2020;1866:165717.
47. Boers J, de Vries EFJ, Glaudemans AWJM, Hospers GAP, Schröder CP. Applications of PET tracers in molecular imaging for breast cancer. Curr Oncol Rep. 2020;22:85.
48. Kömek H, Can C, Güzel Y, Oruç Z, Gündoğan C, Yildirin ÖA, et al. ^{68}Ga-FAPI-04 PET/CT, a new step in breast cancer imaging: a comparative pilot study with the ^{18}F-FDG PET/CT. Ann Nucl Med. 2021;35:744–52.
49. Koolen BB, Vogel WV, Vrancken Peeters MJTFD, Loo CE, Rutgers EJT, Valdés Olmos RA. Molecular imaging in breast cancer: from whole-body PET/CT to dedicated breast PET. J Oncol. 2012;438647
50. Narayanan D, Berg WA. Dedicated breast gamma camera imaging and breast positron emission tomography (breast PET): current status and future directions. PET Clin. 2018;13:363–81.
51. Sasada S, Kimura Y, Masumoto N, Emi A, Kadoya T, Arihiro K, Okada M. Breast cancer detection by dedicated breast positron emission tomography according to the World Health Organization classification of breast tumors. Eur J Surg Oncol. 2021;47:1588–92.
52. Teixeira SC, Ferrér Rebolleda J, Koolen BB, Wesseling J, Jurado S, Stokkel MPM, et al. Evaluation of a hanging breast PET system for primary tumor visualization in patients with stage I-III breast cancer: comparison with standard PET/CT. Am J Roentgenol. 2016b;206:1307–14.
53. Collarino A, Valdés Olmos RA, van der Hoeven AF, Pereira Arias-Bouda LM. Methodological aspects of 99mTc-sestamibi guided biopsy in breast cancer. Clin Transl Imaging. 2016;4:367–76.
54. Conners AL, Maxwell RW, Tortorelli CL, Hruska CB, Rhodes DJ, Boughey JC, et al. Gamma camera breast imaging lexicon. Am J Roentgenol. 2012;199:W767–74.
55. Goldsmith SJ, Parsons W, Guiberteau MJ, Stern LH, Lanzkowsky L, Weigert J, et al. SNM practice guideline for breast scintigraphy with breast-specific Y-cameras 1.0*. J Nucl Med Technol. 2010;38:219–24.
56. Huppe AI, Mehta AK, Brem RF. Molecular breast imaging: a comprehensive review. Semin Ultrasound CT MRI. 2018;39:60–9.
57. Radiology American College. ACR practice parameter for the performance of molecular breast imaging (MBI) using a dedicated gamma camera. https://www.acr.org/-/media/ACR/Files/Practice-Parameters/MBI.pdf (adopted 2017).
58. Heil J, Kuerer HM, Pfob A, Rauch G, Sinn HP, Liefers GJ, et al. Eliminating the breast cancer surgery paradigms after neoadjuvant systemic therapy: current evidence and future challenges. Ann Oncol. 2020;31:61–71.
59. Koolen BB, Donker M, Straver ME, Rutgers EJT, Valdés Olmos RA, Vrancken Peeters MJTFD. Combined PET-CT and axillary lymph node marking with radioactive iodine seeds (Mari procedure) for tailored axillary treatment in node-positive breast cancer after neo-adjuvant therapy. Br J Surg. 2017;104:1188–96.
60. Simons JM, van Nijnatten TJA, van der Pool CC, Luite EJT, Koppert LB, Smidt ML. Diagnostic accuracy of different surgical procedures for axillary staging after neoadjuvant systemic therapy in node-positive breast cancer: a systematic review and meta-analysis. Ann Surg. 2019;269:432–42.
61. Van der Noordaa MEM, van Duijnhoven FH, Straver ME, Groen EJ, Stokkel M, Loo CE, et al. Major reduction in axillary lymph node dissections after neoadjuvant systemic therapy for node positive breast cancer by combining PET/CT and the MARI procedure. Ann Surg Oncol. 2018;25:1512–20.

2 Vulvar Cancer

Elizabeth K. A. Triumbari, Simona M. Fragomeni, Luca Zagaria, Damiano Arciuolo, Valerio Lanni, Vittoria Rufini, and Angela Collarino

2.1 Vulvar Cancer Statistics

Vulvar cancer is a rare gynaecological cancer worldwide, with an estimated incidence of 2.6 and a death rate of 0.6 per 100,000 women per year.

It is most commonly diagnosed among women aged 65–74 years. About 60% of patients are diagnosed with local stage disease (disease confined to the primary site), 28% with spread of disease to regional nodes and 6% with distant metastases.

The 5-year relative survival rate varies from 85.5% for women with localized disease to 50.6% for those with regional disease and to 20.3% for patients with distant disease. The death rate is higher in elderly women [1, 2].

2.2 Aetiology

Human papillomavirus (HPV) infection is the most important risk factor, with HPV-16 and HPV-18 being the most frequent subtypes associated with vulvar cancer. Other risk factors are old age, history of smoking, inflammatory conditions affecting the vulva and chronic immunosuppression [3].

2.3 Anatomy

The vulva is the area between the pubis and the anus antero-posteriorly, and between the ischial tuberosities laterally. It includes the mons pubis, the clitoris, the inner and outer lips, the opening of urethra and vagina, and the perineum (Fig. 2.1).

E. K. A. Triumbari
Section of Nuclear Medicine, University Department of Radiological Sciences and Haematology, Università Cattolica del Sacro Cuore, Rome, Italy

S. M. Fragomeni
Department of Woman and Child Health and Public Health, Vul.Can MDT, Fondazione Policlinico Universitario A. Gemelli IRCCS, Rome, Italy

L. Zagaria · V. Lanni · A. Collarino (✉)
Nuclear Medicine Unit, Fondazione Policlinico Universitario A. Gemelli IRCCS, Rome, Italy
e-mail: angela.collarino@policlinicogemelli.it

D. Arciuolo
Unit of Gynecopathology, Department of Woman and Child Health and Public Health, Fondazione Policlinico Universitario A. Gemelli IRCCS, Rome, Italy

V. Rufini
Section of Nuclear Medicine, University Department of Radiological Sciences and Haematology, Università Cattolica del Sacro Cuore, Rome, Italy

Nuclear Medicine Unit, Fondazione Policlinico Universitario A. Gemelli IRCCS, Rome, Italy

A. Collarino et al. (eds.), *Nuclear Medicine Manual on Gynaecological Cancers and Other Female Malignancies*, https://doi.org/10.1007/978-3-031-05497-6_2

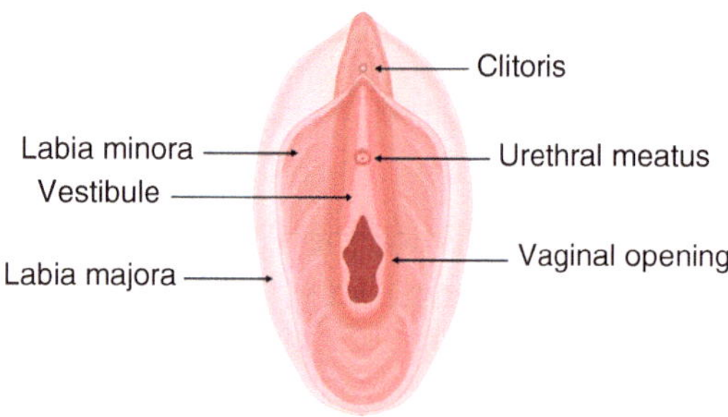

Fig. 2.1 Anatomy of vulva. Courtesy of Vanessa Feudo, Section of Nuclear Medicine, University Department of Radiological Sciences and Haematology, Università Cattolica del Sacro Cuore, Rome, Italy

2.4 Histologic Types

The main histologic type of vulvar cancer is squamous cell carcinoma (SCC) that accounts for about 90% of all vulvar cancers (Fig. 2.2). In particular, there are two pathogenic pathways: HPV infection-related SCC, which occurs in younger women, and HPV-non-related SCC, which mainly occurs in older women.

Other histological types include melanoma, extramammary Paget's disease, adenocarcinoma of Bartholin's gland, verrucous carcinoma, basal cell carcinoma and sarcoma (Fig. 2.2) [4, 5].

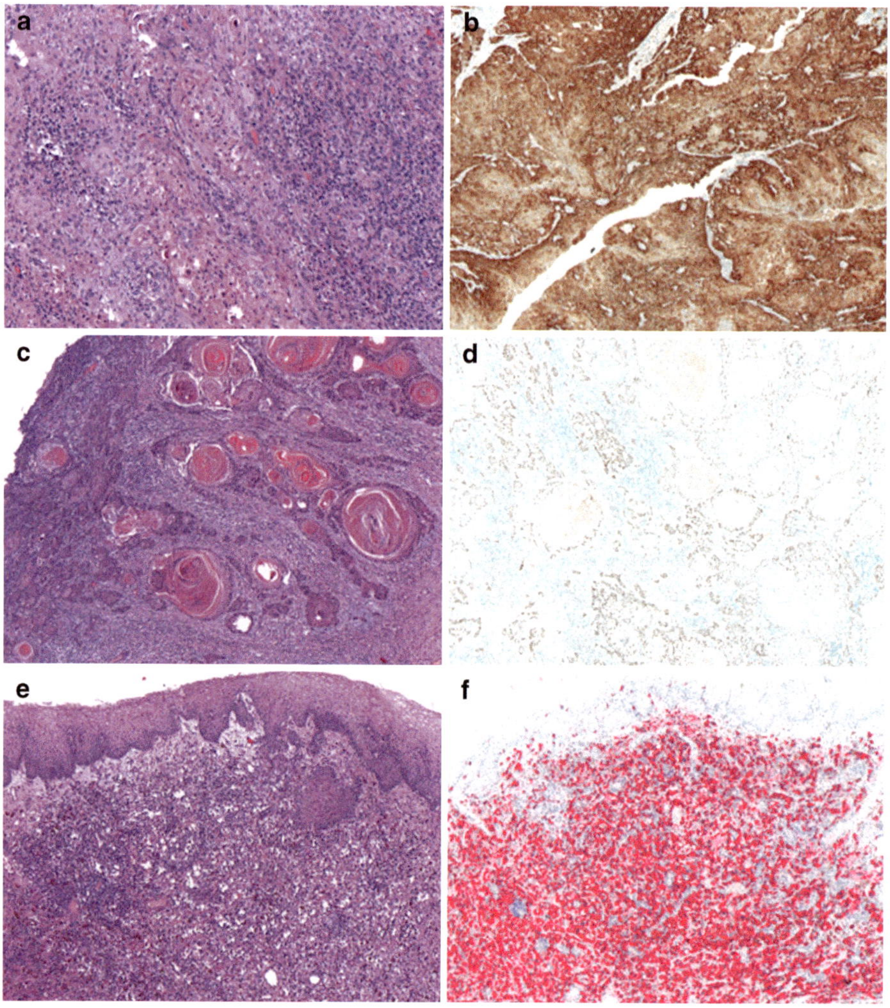

Fig. 2.2 Vulvar squamous cell carcinoma is composed of polygonal cells with abundant eosinophilic cytoplasm without keratin pearls in a desmoplastic stroma (**a**). The pathogenesis of squamous cell carcinoma could be related to HPV infection with a diffuse, block-like staining for p16 (**b**). Vulvar squamous cell carcinoma with keratin pearls in a desmoplastic stroma (**c**) and with a diffuse, block-like staining for p53 (**d**). Vulvar melanoma (**e**) is composed of large cells containing brown melanin pigment in the cytoplasm; the cells show immunoreactivity for Melan-A (**f**)

2.5 Staging

Staging of vulvar cancer is defined according to 2009 FIGO stage (Table 2.1). In case of a multifocal tumour, the target lesion that will address the highest pT stage is the one with the largest diameter or greatest depth of invasion.

Early-stage vulvar cancer concerns 2009 FIGO stage I and smaller stage II, whereas locally advanced vulvar cancer (LAVC) refers to 2009 FIGO stages: larger stage II, stage III and IVA [3, 6].

Table 2.1 2009 FIGO stage

2009 FIGO stage	Description
I	Tumour (T) confined to vulva and/or perineum
IA	T ≤ 2 cm, confined to vulva and/or perineum, with stromal invasion ≤1.0 mm
IB	T > 2 cm, or any size with stromal invasion >1.0 mm, confined to vulva and/or perineum
II	T of any size, extended to lower/distal third of urethra/vagina or to the anus
III	Regional N+ with one or two nodal metastases (N+), each <5 mm or one N+ ≥ 5 mm
IIIA	One or two N+, each <5 mm
	One N+ ≥ 5 mm
	Regional N+ with three or more N+, each <5 mm or two or more N+ ≥ 5 mm or N+ with extranodal extension
IIIB	Three or more N+, each <5 mm, including micrometastases (≤0.2 mm)
	Two or more N+ ≥ 5 mm
IIIC	N+ with extranodal extension
IVA	T of any size, extended to upper/proximal two-thirds of urethra/vagina or to bladder/rectum or fixed to the pelvic bone; fixed or ulcerated regional N+
IVB	Distant metastases, including pelvic N+

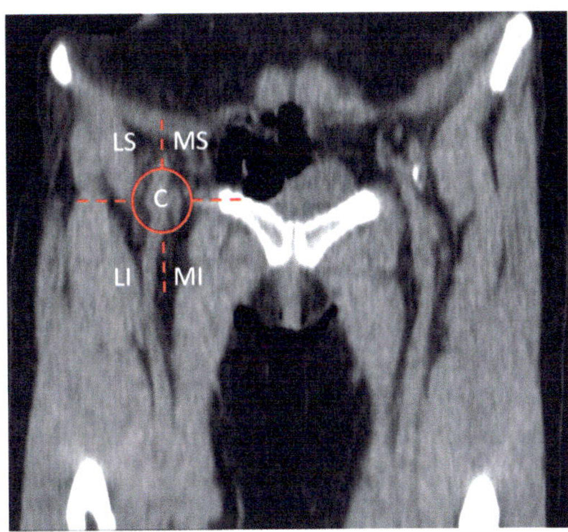

Fig. 2.3 Coronal CT image showing the five Daseler's zones, using the saphenofemoral junction as intersection (red circle). LS: lateral superior zone; MS: medial superior zone; LI: lateral inferior zone; MI: medial inferior zone; C: central zone

2.6 Lymphatic Drainage of the Vulva

Vulvar lymphatic drainage is principally directed to the groin nodes and subsequently to the pelvic nodes (Fig. 2.3). It is unilateral in case of lateral vulvar lesions (located at more than 1–2 cm from the midline) and bilateral in case of midline tumours or tumours located within 1 cm from the midline [7, 8].

2.7 Sentinel Node Biopsy Versus Lymphadenectomy

The presence of nodal involvement is the most important prognostic factor in vulvar cancer patients. The risk of groin lymph node (LN) involvement is low (25–35%) in early-stage disease, thus extensive groin dissection is considered an overtreatment with a high risk of postoperative complications (i.e. wound breakdown, lymphocyst formation and lymphoedema).

Prospective studies support the feasibility of sentinel node biopsy (SNB) in early-stage disease and suggest that extensive groin dissection may be avoided in selected patients.

The histopathological evaluation of sentinel nodes (SNs) with ultra-staging and immunohistochemistry, results in an increased identification of micrometastases and isolated tumour cells, improving nodal staging.

SNB reduces surgical time, length of hospital stays and costs. However, SNB should be only performed in Centres with expertise and training [9–13].

2.8 Sentinel Node Mapping

2.8.1 Indications and Contraindications

Indications and contraindications of SN mapping are summarized in Table 2.2. In case of vulvar melanoma, SNB is indicated when Breslow thickness is assessed between 1 and 4 mm [3, 14].

Table 2.2 Indications and contraindications for SN mapping

Indications	Contraindications
Squamous cell carcinoma (SCC) – Unifocal disease – <4 cm in diameter – >1 mm depth of stromal invasion – Clinically negative nodes (cN0) Vulvar melanoma – 1–4 mm of Breslow thickness	– Previous lymphadenectomy – Previous inguino-pelvic radiotherapy – Nodal invasion (N+)

2.8.2 Radiopharmaceuticals

The radiopharmaceuticals for SN mapping are colloids labelled with Technetium-99 m (^{99m}Tc) are summarized in Table 2.3 [15–17].

2.8.3 Administered Activity and Injection Sites

Local anaesthetic is applied around the vulvar lesion or the scar deriving from a previous diagnostic excision biopsy. After 5–10 min, the radiopharmaceutical is injected intradermally around the tumour edge, using a 25-gauge needle. Four aliquots of 37 MBq of radiotracer are used in the 1-day protocol and 4 aliquots of 74 MBq in the 2-day protocol [15, 18].

2.8.4 Acquisition Protocol

Pelvic dynamic images (Fig. 2.4a) are acquired after radiotracer injection in anterior and posterior projections. Then, early (Fig. 2.4b) and late (Fig. 2.4c) planar images are obtained, respectively, at 15 and 120 min in anterior and lateral views.

After acquisition of late planar images, single photon emission computed tomography with low-dose computed tomography (SPECT/CT) images are obtained (Fig. 2.4d) [15].

2.8.5 Pitfalls in Interpretation

Possible pitfalls are the false-positive SNs due to radioactive contamination or when the SN is met-

Table 2.3 Radiopharmaceuticals for SN mapping

Radiopharmaceuticals	Country	Particle size (nm)	Pros	Cons
^{99m}Tc-nanocolloid	Europe	5–80	Preoperative mapping	Radiation burden
^{99m}Tc-sulphur colloid	United States	100–200 (filtered)		Preoperative injection
^{99m}Tc-antimony trisulphide	Canada/ Australia	3–30		
Indocyanine green (ICG)-^{99m}Tc-nanocolloid	Europe	5–80	Preoperative and intraoperative mapping	

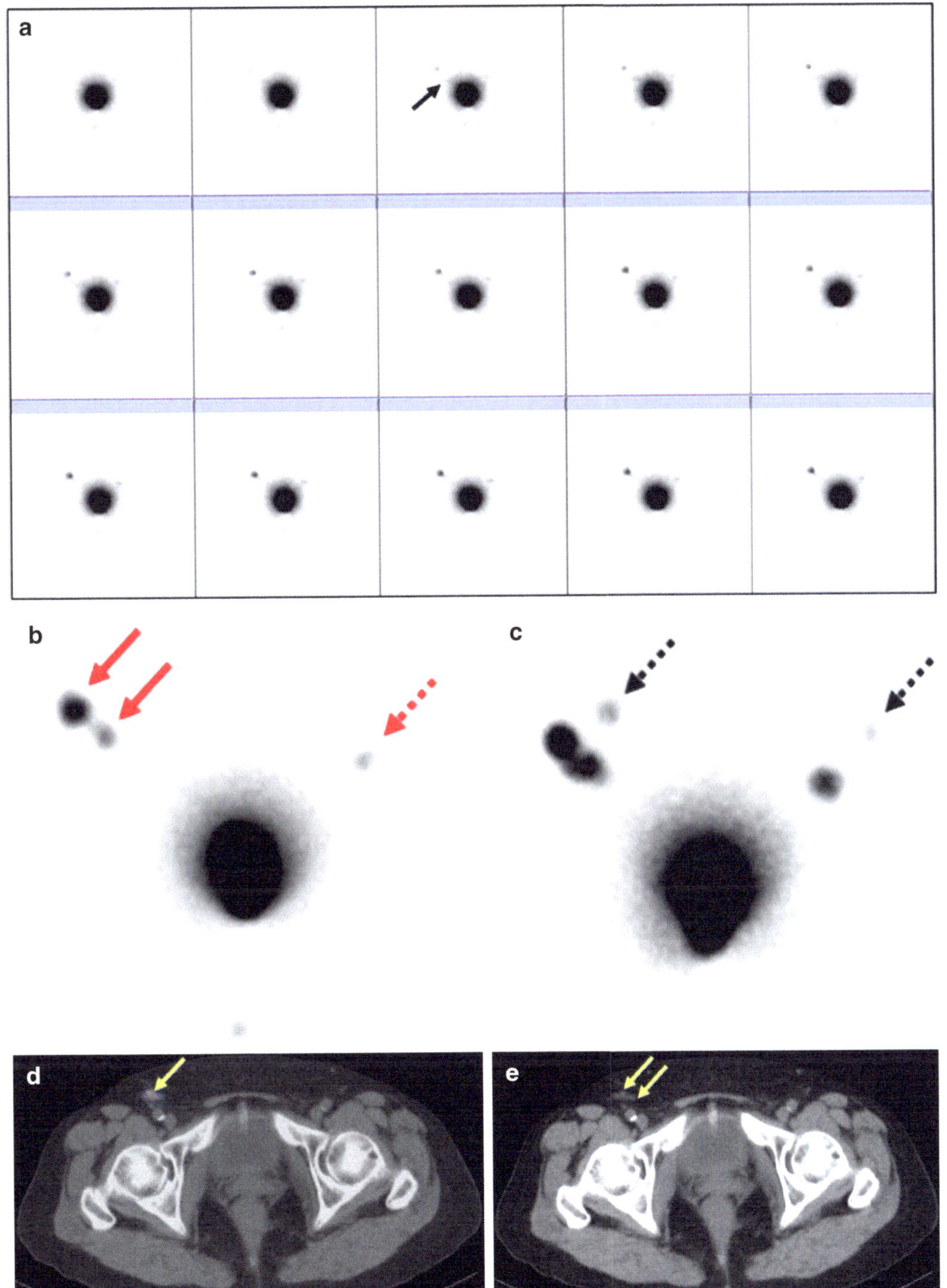

Fig. 2.4 An 83-year-old woman with midline vulvar tumour. Anterior dynamic images (**a**) show bilateral lymphatic drainage with visualization of a right lymphatic duct (arrow). Anterior early image (**b**) shows two SNs in the right groin (red arrows) and one SN in the left groin (red dashed arrow). Anterior late image (**c**) shows one higher-echelon node in the right pelvic region and one higher-echelon node in the left pelvic region (black dashed arrows). Transaxial fused SPECT/CT image (**d**) shows a focal uptake (yellow arrow) in the right groin corresponding to two not enlarged LNs (yellow arrows) on transaxial low-dose CT image (**e**)

astatic, causing lymphatic stasis and bypass of lymphatic flow to other LNs. False-positive SNs due to the radioactive contamination appear as hot spots that can be easily unveiled with SPECT/CT, while imaging of metastatic nodes can be avoided with a careful preoperative anatomical imaging that rules out gross nodal involvement.

Another possible pitfall can be the non-visualization of SNs due to a deep injection, loss of injection fluid, lymphatic stasis or overweight women [19–21].

2.8.6 Utility of SPECT/CT

Preoperative SPECT/CT provides three-dimensional images with better contrast and spatial resolution than planar images, resulting in precise anatomic localization of the SNs and depiction of additional SNs.

Moreover, SPECT/CT images are useful in the detection of SNs localized in uncommon locations and reduces false-positive SNs due to external contamination and presence of radioactivity in enlarged lymphatic vessels [22–25].

2.9 Intraoperative Sentinel Node and Pathological Evaluation

Prior to surgery, an optical tracer, blue dye or ICG, is injected in the same points as the radiotracer injection. In some Centres, mainly in the United States, the optical tracer is the one method applied. If the radiopharmaceutical is injected (intraoperative counting), a gamma probe is used intraoperatively to localize the SNs.

When available, a portable gamma camera could be particularly useful, allowing a better localization of SNs close to the injection site. A fluorescence probe must be used if ICG is injected. After excision of SNs, ex vivo radioactivity of SNs (ex vivo counting) and/or the near-infrared rays of fluorescent SNs are measured.

All excised SNs are sent for haematoxylin and eosin (H&E) staining. If the H&E staining of SNs does not reveal metastases, ultra-staging should be performed to rule out micrometastatic disease. Metastatic SNs guide for a more extensive lymphadenectomy or adjuvant therapy [3, 16, 18].

2.10 PET/CT and Vulvar Cancer

2.10.1 Indications and Contraindications

For clinical routine, ^{18}F-fluorodeoxyglucose (^{18}F-FDG) is used. Indications and contraindications of ^{18}F-FDG positron emission tomography/computed tomography (PET/CT) are summarized in Table 2.4 [3].

2.10.2 Acquisition Protocol

The patient should fast for 6 h before the exam and should have glucose blood levels lower than 200 mg/dl. ^{18}F-FDG is intravenously injected and the patient is hydrated with 500 ml of saline solution to ensure a low concentration of ^{18}F-FDG in the urine. Low-dose CT scan is acquired from the skull to the pelvis for anatomical localization and attenuation correction. PET/CT images are acquired at 60 min (±10 min) after ^{18}F-FDG injection, in the range defined by CT [26].

2.10.3 Image Analysis

For visual analysis, any focus of ^{18}F-FDG uptake at the primary site and at the LN sites and/or distant sites higher than the surrounding background is considered abnormal and interpreted as positive.

Table 2.4 Indications and contraindications for ^{18}F-FDG PET/CT in vulvar cancer

Indications	Contraindications
Staging – Initial workup of T2 or larger tumour or if metastases are suspected Response assessment – If primary treatment was with definitive intent Suspected local or distant recurrence	Glucose blood level > 200 mg/dl

For quantitative analysis, maximum standardized uptake (SUV_{max}) value is the most widely used quantitative parameter. SUV_{max} is defined as the hottest voxel within the volume of interest (VOI). Also, SUV_{peak} (mean SUV of a sphere of 12 mm diameter centred on SUV_{max}) and SUV_{mean} (mean SUV within the tumour) are frequently used.

Volumetric PET parameters are metabolic tumour volume (MTV), which represents the volume of functioning cells, and total lesion glycolysis (TLG = MTV x SUV_{mean}), which combines the metabolic and volumetric information of the entire tumour (Fig. 2.5).

2.10.4 Pitfalls in Interpretation

Possible pitfalls in interpretation are due to false-positive (Fig. 2.6) inflammatory LNs, due to the presence of activated macrophages and other inflammatory cells in the drainage sites of the vulvar region, especially following biopsy, medical procedures or shaving; or false-negative LNs, due to presence of micrometastases or necrosis (Fig. 2.7) [27].

SUV_{max}	31.9
SUV_{peak}	18.1/size 1 cm^3
SUV_{mean}	19.9
MTV	2.0 cm^3
TLG	38.2
Threshold	12.7/40%

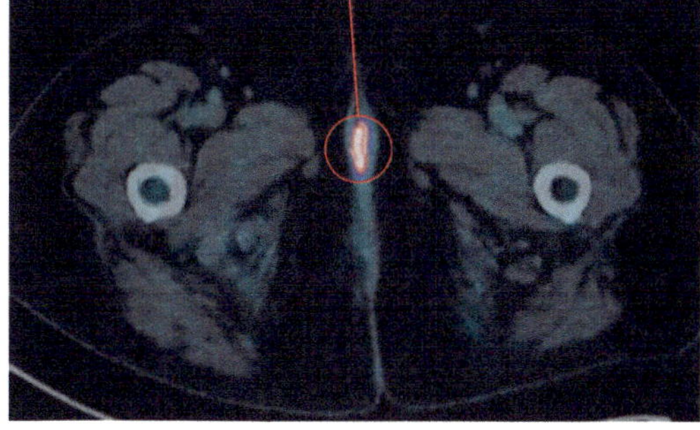

Fig. 2.5 Quantitative parameters of a primary vulvar tumour lesion

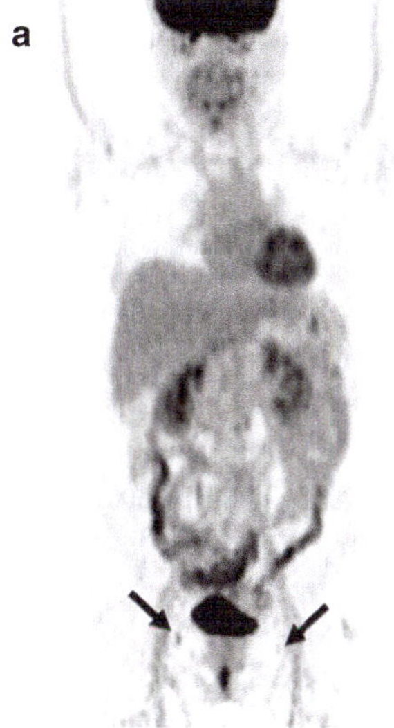

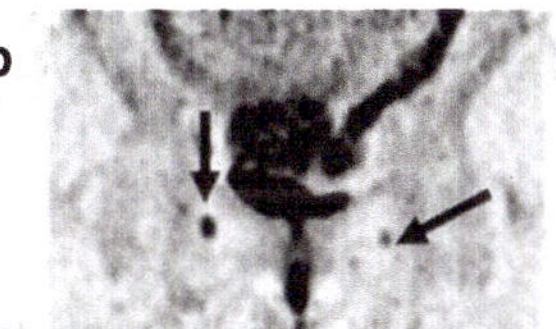

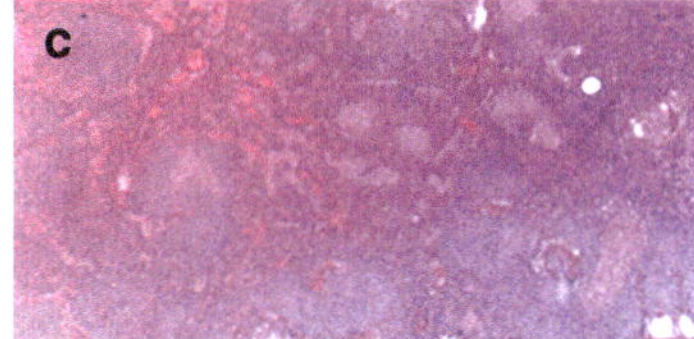

Fig. 2.6 A 60-year-old woman with midline tumour. Maximum intensity projection (MIP, **a**) of standard ^{18}F-FDG PET/CT image showing focal uptake in right groin (SUV_{max} 3.5) and in left groin (SUV_{max} 2) (arrows). Maximum intensity projection (MIP, **b**) of delayed scan showing an increase of focal uptake in the right groin (SUV_{max} 6.39) and in the left groin (SUV_{max} 3.41). Pathologic examination (**c**) showed no metastatic LNs in either groin. Courtesy of Collarino A, Garganese G, Valdés Olmos RA, Stefanelli A, Perotti G, Mirk P, et al. Evaluation of Dual-Timepoint 18F-FDG PET/CT Imaging for Lymph Node Staging in Vulvar Cancer. J Nucl Med. 2017;58(12):1913–1918. https://doi.org/10.2967/jnumed.117.194332

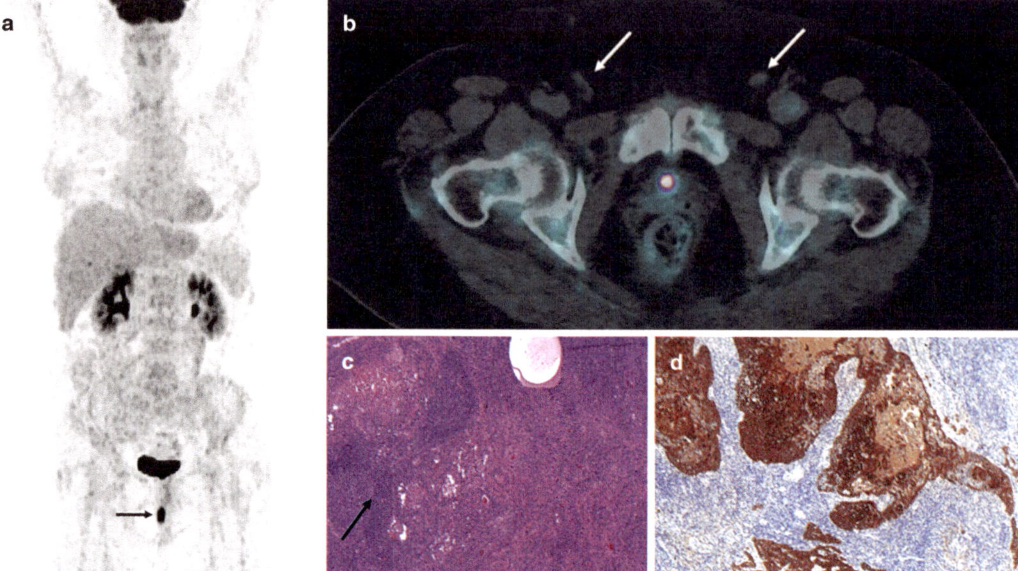

Fig. 2.7 A 69-year-old woman with untreated invasive midline vulvar squamous cell carcinoma. Maximum intensity projection image (MIP, **a**) showing no ^{18}F-FDG uptake other than at the primary tumour (arrow). Transaxial fused PET/CT image (**b**) showing no uptake in groin nodes (white arrows). Pathologic examination revealed metastasis of 2 mm in one of two SNs in the left groin (**c**, arrow; **d**, the neoplastic cells are highlighted by the immunohistochemical test for CK AE1/AE3) and metastasis of 2.5 mm in one of the two SNs in the right groin

2.11 Diagnostic Utility of PET/CT

2.11.1 Staging and Therapy Planning

According to international guidelines, PET/CT is recommended for vulvar cancer staging, in particular for LN and distant metastases (Fig. 2.8), as primary tumour extent (T-staging) is more accurately carried out with magnetic resonance (MR).

Preoperative PET/CT has a moderate pooled sensitivity (0.76, 95%CI, 0.57–0.94) and reasonable specificity (0.88, 95%CI, 0.82–0.94) in detecting metastatic groin nodes using a qualitative (visual) analysis. This resulted in a good pooled negative predictive value (NPV) (0.92; 95% CI: 0.86–0.97) that could justify a less invasive surgical treatment in early-stage vulvar cancer patients (cN0) currently unfit for SNB. However, it should be kept in mind that PET/CT's spatial resolution is not adequate to reliably detect micrometastatic disease (Fig. 2.7) or the presence of necrosis and subsequent loss of ^{18}F-FDG uptake in the examined LNs. It is expected that new digital PET systems with small voxel reconstruction will allow the detection of small metastatic LNs, thus improving the diagnostic results in cN0 vulvar cancer patients.

On the other hand, the positive predictive value (PPV) resulting from a recent meta-analysis was 70%. Therefore, a PET-positive groin node needs to be interpreted with caution due to visualization of inflammatory nodes and should not immediately justify an aggressive course of management. Unlike other neoplasms, specificity and PPV of PET/CT in detecting groin metastases do not improve at delayed PET/CT (at 3 h from ^{18}F-FDG injection) (Fig. 2.6).

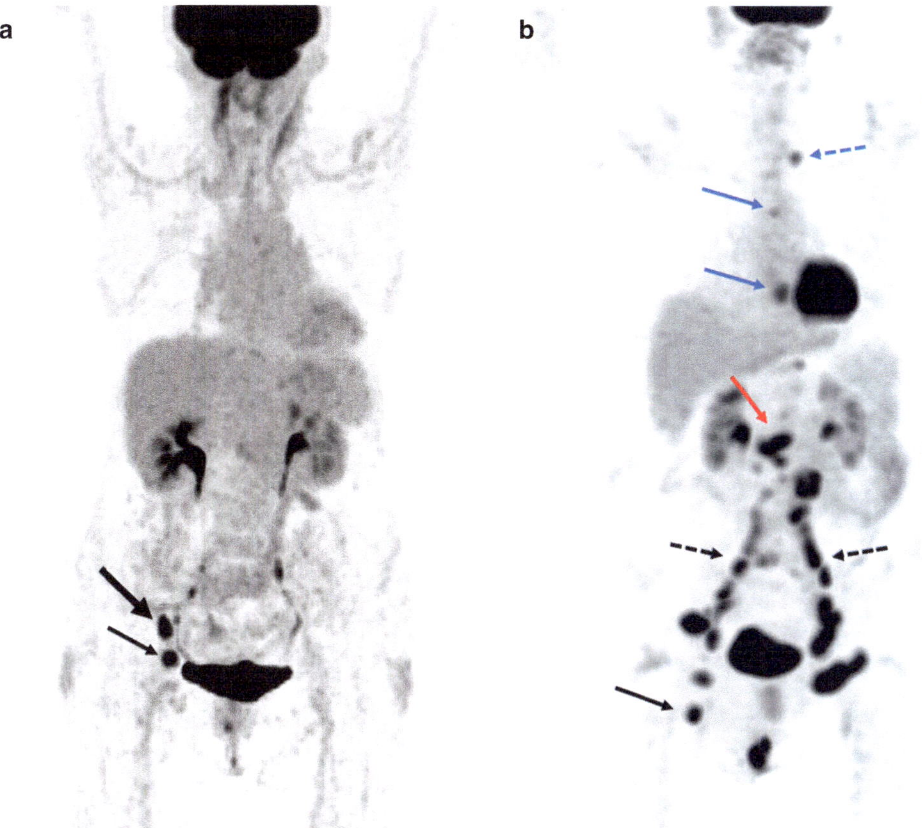

Fig. 2.8 A 76-year-old woman with vulvar cancer, diagnosed on excisional biopsy. Maximum intensity projection image (MIP, **a**) showing two focal areas of ^{18}F-FDG uptake corresponding to two right pelvic nodes (arrows). An 80-year-old woman with untreated vulvar squamous cell carcinoma. Maximum intensity projection image (MIP, **b**) showing multiple focal areas of ^{18}F-FDG uptake corresponding to disease spread to the right groin (black arrow), pelvic (black dashed arrows) and abdominal peri-aortic nodes (red arrow), para-oesophageal (blue arrows) and left retro-clavicular nodes (blue dashed arrow)

As for the detection of metastatic pelvic nodes or distant metastases (i.e. lung, bone and liver), PET/CT showed high sensitivity and NPV (100%) and a 57% specificity and 33% PPV on a patient-based analysis [28–32].

2.11.2 Response Assessment

In LAVC patients, ^{18}F-FDG PET/CT performed at baseline and at 3 months post completion of therapy is routinely used for response assessment. Baseline (pre-treatment) PET/CT helps to tailor treatment, while post-therapy PET/CT is useful to assess metabolic response (Fig. 2.9) and to predict prognosis.

In particular, partial metabolic response (PMR) or progressive disease (PD) on post-therapy PET/CT is associated with worse locoregional control and overall survival than complete metabolic response [33].

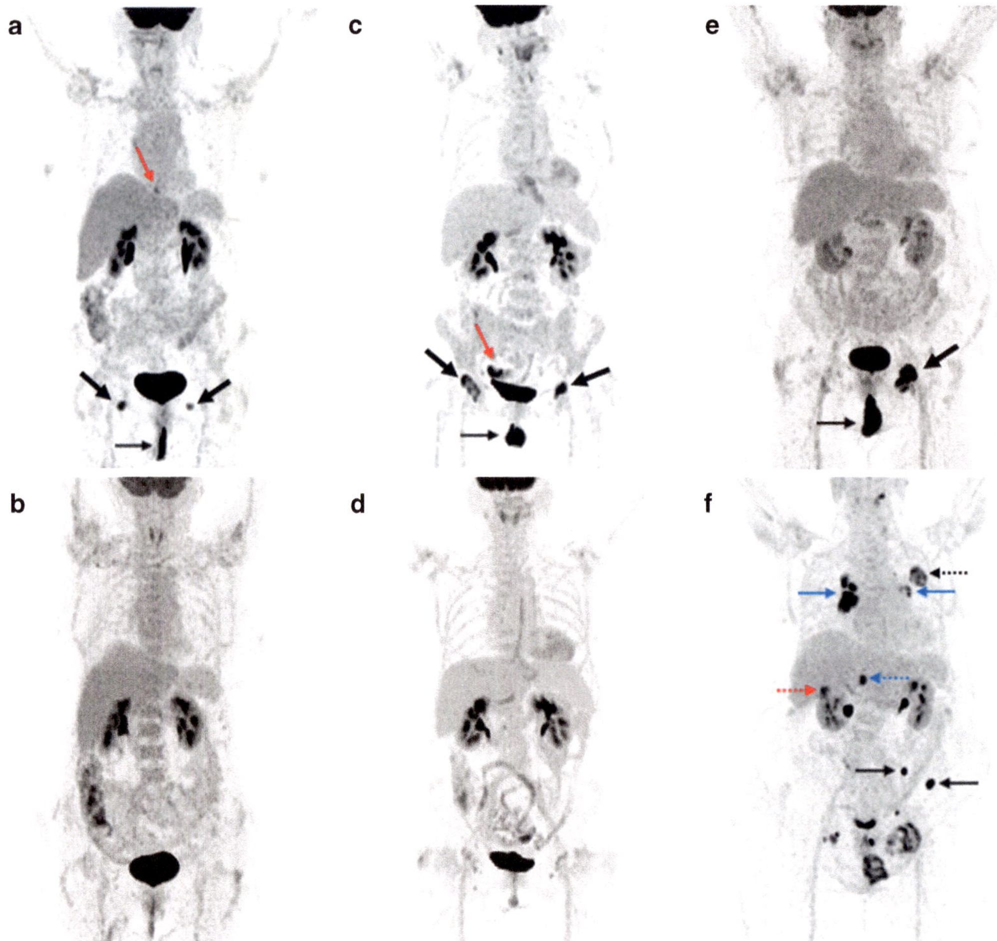

Fig. 2.9 An 83-year-old woman with vulvar squamous cell carcinoma. Maximum intensity projection image (MIP, **a**) showing ^{18}F-FDG uptake corresponding to the primary tumour (thin arrow) and to bilateral groin nodes (thick arrows), non-specific focal uptake is detected in the lower third of the oesophagus (red arrow); maximum intensity projection images (MIP, **b**) showing complete response to radio-chemotherapy. A 72-year-old woman with vulvar squamous cell carcinoma. Maximum intensity projection image (MIP, **c**) showing ^{18}F-FDG uptake corresponding to the primary tumour (thin arrow), to bilateral groin nodes (thick arrows), non-specific intestinal ^{18}F-FDG uptake (red arrow); maximum intensity projection image (MIP, **d**) showing partial response to the radio-chemotherapy. An 87-year-old woman with vulvar squamous cell carcinoma. Maximum intensity projection image (MIP, **e**) showing ^{18}F-FDG uptake corresponding to the primary tumour (thin arrow) and to large left groin nodes (thick arrow); maximum intensity projection image (MIP, **f**) showing disease progression after radio-chemotherapy at inguinal (partially necrotic nodes), pelvic, abdominal (blue dashed arrow) and supra-diaphragmatic nodes (pulmonary hila, blue arrows), liver (red dashed arrow), left lung (black dashed arrow) and bone metastases (black arrows)

2.11.3 Restaging for Suspected Recurrence

Disease recurrence occurs in approximately one-third of patients within the first 1–2 years after therapy. The sites of recurrence are vulva, inguinal nodes, pelvic nodes and distant metastases. The survival rate after recurrence is low and the cure efficacy is minimal.

In case of suspected recurrence, PET/CT has a high sensitivity (100%, 95%CI, 93–100%) and specificity (92%, 95%CI, 62–100%) in detection of nodal and distant relapse (Fig. 2.10) [34].

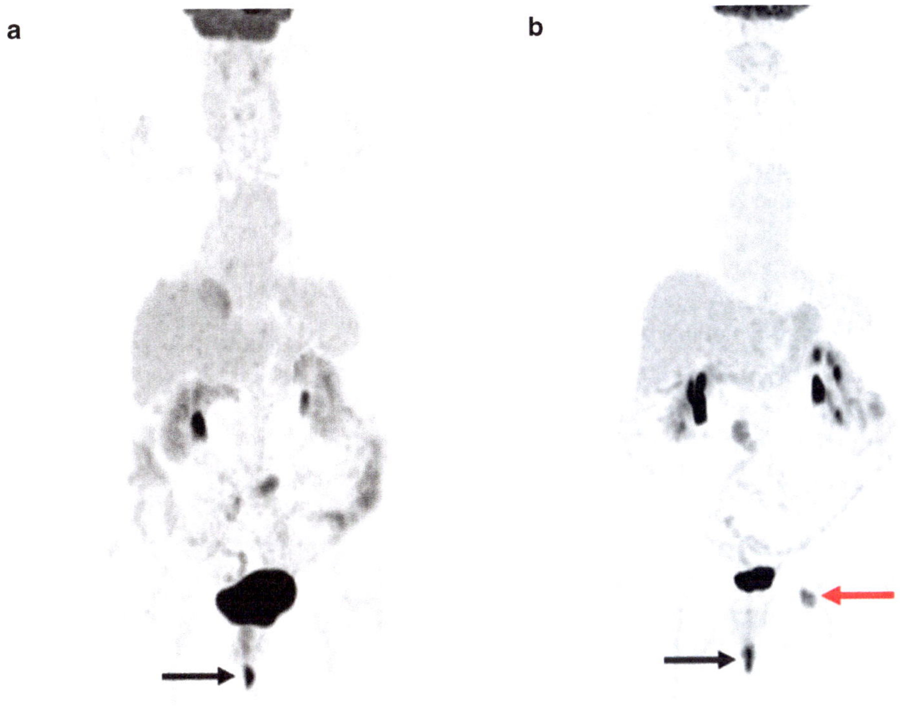

Fig. 2.10 A 70-year-old woman with vulvar cancer. Maximum intensity projection image (MIP, **a**) of staging PET/CT showing ^{18}F-FDG uptake corresponding to the primary tumour (black arrow); the patient was then treated with radical vulvectomy. Maximum intensity projection image (MIP, **b**) of restaging PET/CT for a cytological finding of local recurrence showing ^{18}F-FDG uptake in the vulvar region (local recurrence, black arrow) and a focal ^{18}F-FDG uptake in the left groin region (groin recurrence, red arrow)

2.12 Vaginal Cancer

Vaginal cancer is a very rare tumour with an incidence rate of 1 per 100,000/year. HPV infection is the most important risk factor. The 5-year survival rates vary from 67% for women with localized disease, to 52% for those with regional disease and to 19% for patients with distant disease.

The main histological type of vaginal cancer is SCC, which accounts for about 90% of all vaginal cancers. Other histological types include adenocarcinoma, sarcoma and melanoma.

Staging of vaginal cancer is defined according to 2012 FIGO stage (Table 2.5).

The lymphatic drainage of the upper vagina is directed to the pelvic and para-aortic nodes, while the lymphatic drainage of the lower vagina is directed to the inguino-femoral nodes.

Since the risk of metastatic LNs is low in early-stage disease, pelvic and groin dissection may be spared in absence of proven metastatic nodes. Therefore, SNB could be useful in early-stage cases. The sentinel node mapping is similar to that described for vulvar cancer, apart from the radiotracer injection sites that for vaginal cancer are at 3, 6, 9 and 12 o'clock around the primary vaginal tumour.

PET/CT is useful in evaluating recurrent disease and distant metastases (Fig. 2.11) whereas the extent of local tumour infiltration is carried out with MR [35–39].

Table 2.5 2012 FIGO stage

2012 FIGO stage	Description
IA	Tumour (T) $\leq$ 2 cm, confined to vagina
IB	T > 2 cm, confined to vagina
IIA	T $\leq$ 2 cm, extended to vaginal wall
IIB	T > 2 cm, extended to vaginal wall
III	T of any size, extended to pelvic wall/ hydro-nephrosis/pelvic or groin N+
IVA	T extended to bladder or rectum or out of pelvis, any N
IVB	T of any size, distant metastases (i.e. lung, liver or bone)

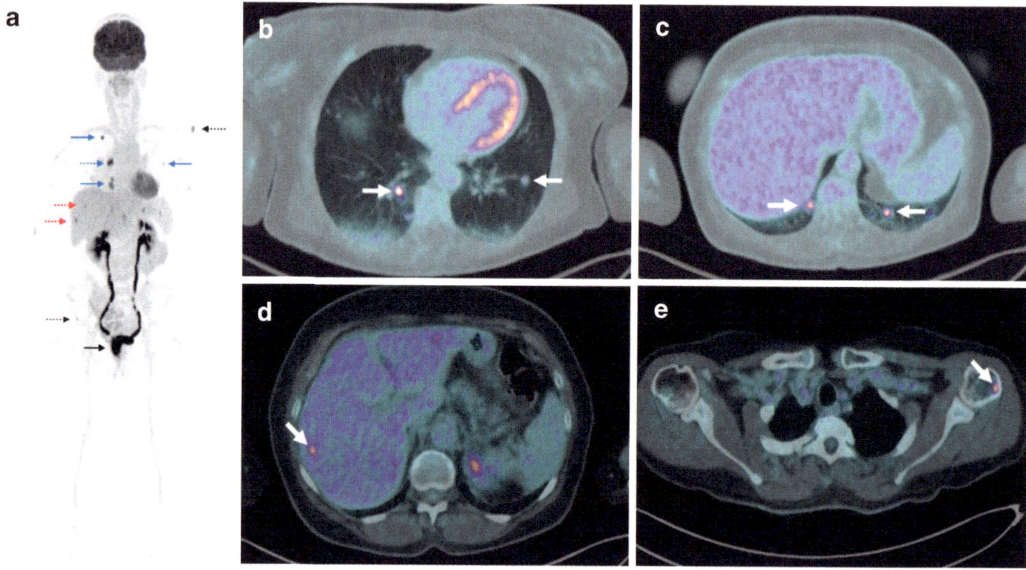

Fig. 2.11 A 53-year-old woman with diagnosis of vaginal melanoma. Maximum intensity projection images (MIP, **a**) showing intense ^{18}F-FDG uptake corresponding to the primary tumour (black arrow), multiple bilateral lung metastases (blue arrows), right pulmonary hilum lymphadenomegaly (blue dashed arrow), multiple liver (red dashed arrows) and bone (black dashed arrows) lesions. Transverse fused PET/CT images showing some of the bilateral lung nodules (**b**, **c**), a liver lesion (**d**) and a left proximal humerus lesion (**e**)

References

1. Siegel RL, Miller KD, Jemal A. Cancer statistics, 2020. CA Cancer J Clin. 2020;70(1):7–30. https://doi.org/10.3322/caac.21590.
2. SEER Cancer Stat Facts: Vulvar Cancer. National Cancer Institute, Bethesda https://seer.cancer.gov/statfacts/html/vulva.html. Accessed Jan 2021.
3. Abu-Rustum NR, Yashar CM, Bradley K, Campos SM, Chon HS, Chu C, et al. Vulvar cancer (Squamous Cell Carcinoma): Version 3.2021. In: NCCN Clinical Practice Guidelines in Oncology (NCCN guidelines); 2021. https://www.nccn.org/professionals/physician_gls/pdf/vulvar.pdf. Accessed 15 Sept 2021.
4. Hacker NF, Eifel PJ, van der Velden J. Cancer of the vulva. Int J Gynaecol Obstet. 2012;119(2):S90–6. https://doi.org/10.1016/S0020-7292(12)60021-6.
5. Del Pino M, Rodriguez-Carunchio L, Ordi J. Pathways of vulvar intraepithelial neoplasia and squamous cell carcinoma. Histopathology. 2013;62(1):161–75. https://doi.org/10.1111/his.12034.
6. Hacker NF. Revised FIGO staging for carcinoma of the vulva. Int J Gynaecol Obstet. 2009;105(2):105–6. https://doi.org/10.1016/j.ijgo.2009.02.011.
7. Daseler EH, Anson BJ, Reimann AF. Radical excision of the inguinal and iliac lymph glands; a study based upon 450 anatomical dissections and upon supportive clinical observations. Surg Gynecol Obstet. 1948;87(6):679–94.
8. Iversen T, Aas M. Lymph drainage from the vulva. Gynecol Oncol. 1983;16(2):179–89. https://doi.org/10.1016/0090-8258(83)90092-6.
9. Burger MPM, Hollema H, Emanuels AG, Krans M, Pras E, Bouma J. The importance of the groin node status for the survival of T1 and T2 Vulval carcinoma patients. Gynecol Oncol. 1995;57(3):327–34. https://doi.org/10.1006/gyno.1995.1151.
10. Gaarenstroom KN, Kenter GG, Trimbos JB, Agous I, Amant F, Peters AAW, et al. Postoperative complications after vulvectomy and inguinofemoral lymphadenectomy using separate groin incisions. Int J Gynecol Cancer. 2003;13(4):522–7. https://doi.org/10.1046/j.1525-1438.2003.13304.x.
11. Levenback CF, Ali S, Coleman RL, Gold MA, Fowler JM, Judson PL, et al. Lymphatic mapping and sentinel lymph node biopsy in women with squamous cell carcinoma of the vulva: a gynecologic oncology group study. J Clin Oncol. 2012;30(31):3786–91. https://doi.org/10.1200/JCO.2011.41.2528.
12. Oonk MH, van Hemel BM, Hollema H, de Hullu JA, Ansink AC, Vergote I, et al. Size of sentinel-node metastasis and chances of non-sentinel-node involvement and survival in early stage vulvar cancer: results from GROINSS-V, a multicentre observational study. Lancet Oncol. 2010;11(7):646–52. https://doi.org/10.1016/S1470-2045(10)70104-2.
13. Van der Zee AGJ, Oonk MH, De Hullu JA, Ansink AC, Vergote I, Verheijen RH, et al. Sentinel node dissection is safe in the treatment of early-stage vulvar cancer. J Clin Oncol. 2008;26(6):884–9. https://doi.org/10.1200/JCO.2007.14.0566.
14. de Hullu JA, Hollema H, Hoekstra HJ, Piers DA, Mourits MJ, Aalders JG, et al. Vulvar melanoma: is there a role for sentinel lymph node biopsy? Cancer. 2002;94(2):486–91. https://doi.org/10.1002/cncr.10230.
15. Giammarile F, Bozkurt MF, Cibula D, Pahisa J, Oyen WJ, Paredes P, et al. The EANM clinical and technical guidelines for lymphoscintigraphy and sentinel node localization in gynaecological cancers. Eur J Nucl Med Mol Imaging. 2014;41(7):1463–77. https://doi.org/10.1007/s00259-014-2732-8.
16. Mathéron HM, van den Berg NS, Brouwer OR, Kleinjan GH, van Driel WJ, Trum JW, et al. Multimodal surgical guidance towards the sentinel node in vulvar cancer. Gynecol Oncol. 2013;131(3):720–5. https://doi.org/10.1016/j.ygyno.2013.09.007.
17. Verbeek FP, Tummers QR, Rietbergen DD, Peters AA, Schaafsma BE, van de Velde CJ, et al. Sentinel lymph node biopsy in vulvar Cancer using combined radioactive and fluorescence guidance. Int J Gynecol Cancer. 2015;25(6):1086–93. https://doi.org/10.1097/IGC.0000000000000419.
18. Collarino A, Fuoco V, Garganese G, Pereira Arias-Bouda LM, Perotti G, Manca G, et al. Lymphoscintigraphy and sentinel lymph node biopsy in vulvar carcinoma: update from a European expert panel. Eur J Nucl Med Mol Imaging. 2020;47(5):1261–74. https://doi.org/10.1007/s00259-019-04650-8.
19. Bluemel C, Campos F, Collarino A, Cramer A, Dik S, Giordano A, et al. Case reports. In: Herrmann K, Nieweg O, Povoski S, editors. Radioguided surgery. Springer: Cham; 2016. p. 483–94. https://doi.org/10.1007/978-3-319-26051-8_29.
20. de Hullu JA, Oonk MH, Ansink AC, Hollema H, Jager PL, van der Zee AG. Pitfalls in the sentinel lymph node procedure in vulvar cancer. Gynecol Oncol. 2004;94(1):10–5. https://doi.org/10.1016/j.ygyno.2004.02.031.
21. Fons G, ter Rahe B, Sloof G, de Hullu J, van der Velden J. Failure in the detection of the sentinel lymph node with a combined technique of radioactive tracer and blue dye in a patient with cancer of the vulva and a single positive lymph node. Gynecol Oncol. 2004;92(3):981–4. https://doi.org/10.1016/j.ygyno.2003.12.006.
22. Belhocine TZ, Prefontaine M, Lanvin D, Bertrand M, Rachinsky I, Ettler H, et al. Added-value of SPECT/CT to lymphatic mapping and sentinel lymphadenectomy in gynaecological cancers. Am J Nucl Med Mol Imaging. 2013;3(2):182–93.
23. Beneder C, Fuechsel FG, Krause T, Kuhn A, Mueller MD. The role of 3D fusion imaging in sentinel lymphadenectomy for vulvar cancer. Gynecol Oncol. 2008;109(1):76–80. https://doi.org/10.1016/j.ygyno.2007.11.045.
24. Klapdor R, Länger F, Gratz KF, Hillemanns P, Hertel H. SPECT/CT for SLN dissection in vulvar cancer: improved SLN detection and dissection by preop-

erative three-dimensional anatomical localisation. Gynecol Oncol. 2015;138(3):590–6. https://doi.org/10.1016/j.ygyno.2015.06.011.

25. Kraft O, Havel M. Detection of sentinel lymph nodes in gynecologic tumours by planar scintigraphy and SPECT/CT. Mol Imaging Radionucl Ther. 2012;21(2):47–55. https://doi.org/10.4274/Mirt.236.
26. Boellaard R, Delgado-Bolton R, Oyen WJ, Giammarile F, Tatsch K, Eschner W, et al. FDG PET/CT: EANM procedure guidelines for tumour imaging: version 2.0. Eur J Nucl Med Mol Imaging. 2015;42(2):328–54. https://doi.org/10.1007/s00259-014-2961-x.
27. Perry LJ, Guralp O, Al-Niaimi A, Zucker NA, Kushner DM. False positive PET-CT scan and clinical examination in a patient with locally advanced vulvar cancer. Gynecol Oncol Case Rep. 2013;4:29–31. https://doi.org/10.1016/j.gynor.2012.12.009.
28. Cheng G, Torigian DA, Zhuang H, Alavi A. When should we recommend use of dual time-point and delayed time-point imaging techniques in FDG PET? Eur J Nucl Med Mol Imaging. 2013;40(5):779–87. https://doi.org/10.1007/s00259-013-2343-9.
29. Collarino A, Garganese G, Valdés Olmos RA, Stefanelli A, Perotti G, Mirk P, et al. Evaluation of dual-timepoint 18F-FDG PET/CT imaging for lymph node staging in vulvar cancer. J Nucl Med. 2017;58(12):1913–8. https://doi.org/10.2967/jnumed.117.194332.
30. Lin G, Chen CY, Liu FY, Yang LY, Huang HJ, Huang YT, et al. Computed tomography, magnetic resonance imaging and FDG positron emission tomography in the management of vulvar malignancies. Eur Radiol. 2015;25(5):1267–78. https://doi.org/10.1007/s00330-014-3530-1.
31. Rufini V, Garganese G, Ieria FP, Pasciuto T, Fragomeni SM, Gui B, et al. Diagnostic performance of preoperative [18F]FDG-PET/CT for lymph node staging in vulvar cancer: a large single-Centre study. Eur J Nucl Med Mol Imaging. 2021;48(10):3303–14. https://doi.org/10.1007/s00259-021-05257-8.
32. Triumbari EKA, de Koster EJ, Rufini V, Fragomeni SM, Garganese G, Collarino A. 18F-FDG PET and 18F-FDG PET/CT in vulvar cancer: a systematic review and meta-analysis. Clin Nucl Med. 2021;46(2):125–32. https://doi.org/10.1097/RLU.0000000000003411.
33. Rao YJ, Hassanzadeh C, Chundury A, Hui C, Siegel BA, Dehdashti F, et al. Association of post-treatment positron emission tomography with locoregional control and survival after radiation therapy for squamous cell carcinoma of the vulva. Radiother Oncol. 2017;122(3):445–51. https://doi.org/10.1016/j.radonc.2016.12.019.
34. Albano D, Bonacina M, Savelli G, Ferro P, Busnardo E, Gianolli L, et al. Clinical and prognostic ^{18}F-FDG PET/CT role in recurrent vulvar cancer: a multicentric experience. Jpn J Radiol. 2021; https://doi.org/10.1007/s11604-021-01173-x.
35. Descheemaeker V, Garin E, Morcel K, Lesimple T, Burtin F, Levêque J. Radioisotopic location of the sentinel node in vaginal mucous melanoma before laparoscopic sampling. Surg Laparosc Endosc Percutan Tech. 2008;18(2):195–6. https://doi.org/10.1097/SLE.0b013e318169290c.
36. Dhar KK, Das N, Brinkman DA, Beynon JL, Woolas RP. Utility of sentinel node biopsy in vulvar and vaginal melanoma: report of two cases and review of the literature. Int J Gynecol Cancer. 2007;17(3):720–3. https://doi.org/10.1111/j.1525-1438.2007.00885.x.
37. Frumovitz M, Gayed IW, Jhingran A, Euscher ED, Coleman RL, Ramirez PT, et al. Lymphatic mapping and sentinel lymph node detection in women with vaginal cancer. Gynecol Oncol. 2008;108(3):478–81. https://doi.org/10.1016/j.ygyno.2007.12.001.
38. Robertson NL, Hricak H, Sonoda Y, et al. The impact of FDG-PET/CT in the management of patients with vulvar and vaginal cancer. Gynecol Oncol. 2016;140(3):420–4.
39. van Dam P, Sonnemans H, van Dam PJ, Verkinderen L, Dirix LY. Sentinel node detection in patients with vaginal carcinoma. Gynecol Oncol. 2004;92(1):89–92. https://doi.org/10.1016/j.ygyno.2003.08.006.

Cervical Cancer

3

Vanessa Feudo, Angela Collarino, Damiano Arciuolo, Margherita Lorusso, Gabriella Ferrandina, and Vittoria Rufini

3.1 Cervical Cancer Statistics

Cervical cancer is the fourth most frequent cancer in women worldwide, with an incidence rate of 7.4 and a death rate of 2.2 per 100,000 women per year.

It is most commonly diagnosed among women aged 35–44 years, while the death rate is higher among women aged 55–64 years.

Forty-four percent of women with cervical cancer are diagnosed with local stage disease (disease confined to the primary site), 36% with spread of disease to regional nodes and 16% with distant metastases.

The 5-year relative survival rate varies from 91.9% in women with localized disease to 58.2% in those with regional disease and to 17.6% for patients with distant disease [1, 2].

3.2 Aetiology

Human papillomavirus (HPV) infection is the most important risk factor, with HPV-16 and HPV-18 being the most frequent subtypes associated with cervical cancer. Other risk factors are history of smoking, the use of oral contraceptives, certain autoimmune diseases and chronic immunosuppression [3, 4].

3.3 Anatomy

The uterine cervix is the most distal part of the uterus that links the uterine cavity to the vagina (Fig. 3.1). The uterine cervix is divided into the ectocervix and endocervix.

V. Feudo
Section of Nuclear Medicine, University Department of Radiological Sciences and Haematology, Università Cattolica del Sacro Cuore, Rome, Italy

A. Collarino (✉) · M. Lorusso
Nuclear Medicine Unit, Fondazione Policlinico Universitario A. Gemelli IRCCS, Rome, Italy
e-mail: angela.collarino@policlinicogemelli.it

D. Arciuolo
Unit of Gynecopathology, Department of Woman and Child Health and Public Health, Fondazione Policlinico Universitario A. Gemelli IRCCS, Rome, Italy

G. Ferrandina
Institute of Obstetrics and Gynaecology, Università Cattolica del Sacro Cuore, Rome, Italy

Gynecologic Oncology Unit, Fondazione Policlinico Universitario A. Gemelli IRCCS, Rome, Italy

V. Rufini
Section of Nuclear Medicine, University Department of Radiological Sciences and Haematology, Università Cattolica del Sacro Cuore, Rome, Italy

Nuclear Medicine Unit, Fondazione Policlinico Universitario A. Gemelli IRCCS, Rome, Italy

A. Collarino et al. (eds.), *Nuclear Medicine Manual on Gynaecological Cancers and Other Female Malignancies*, https://doi.org/10.1007/978-3-031-05497-6_3

The ectocervix is the most distal part of the cervix. The external *os* is the opening of the ectocervix into the upper vagina. The ectocervix is lined by squamous cells.

The endocervix (endocervical canal) is the more proximal and inner part of the cervix. The internal *os* is the opening of the endocervix into uterine cavity. The endocervix is lined by glandular cells.

3.4 Histologic Types

The main histologic type of cervical cancer is squamous cell carcinoma (SCC) that accounts for about 80% of all cervical cancers (Fig. 3.2).

Other histologic types are adenocarcinoma, adenosquamous carcinoma, small cell and large cell neuroendocrine carcinoma (Fig. 3.2) [5, 6].

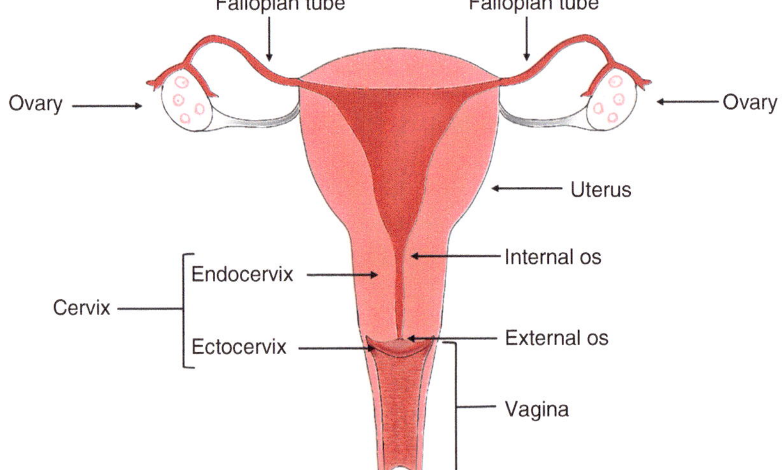

Fig. 3.1 Anatomy of uterine cervix

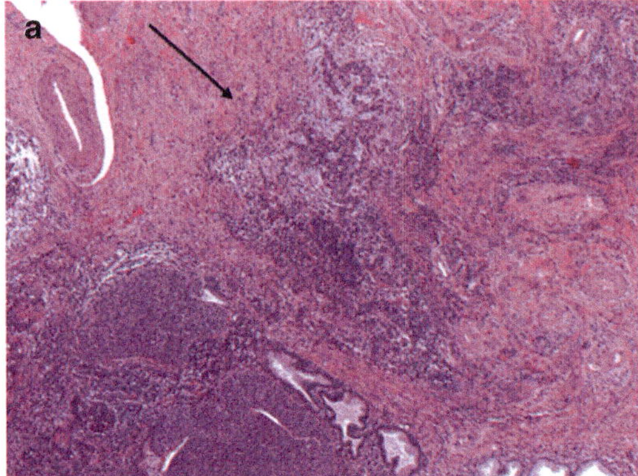

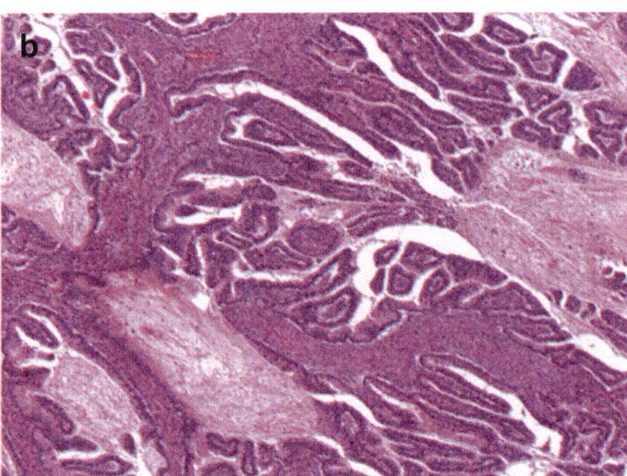

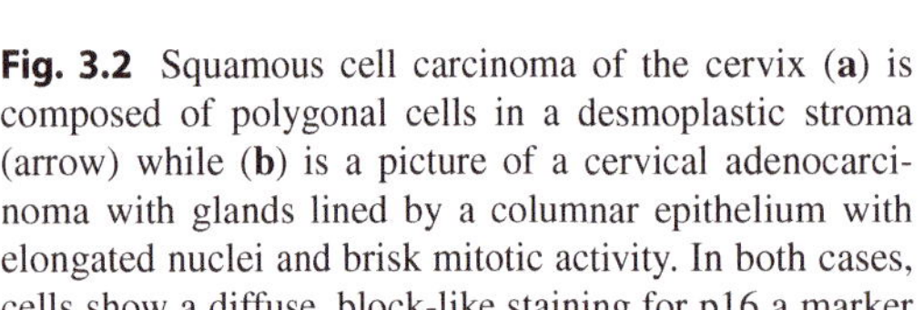

Fig. 3.2 Squamous cell carcinoma of the cervix (**a**) is composed of polygonal cells in a desmoplastic stroma (arrow) while (**b**) is a picture of a cervical adenocarcinoma with glands lined by a columnar epithelium with elongated nuclei and brisk mitotic activity. In both cases, cells show a diffuse, block-like staining for p16 a marker used by pathologists in the evaluation of HPV-related lesions (**c**, **d**). Neuroendocrine carcinoma of the cervix (**e**) is arranged in solid nests, trabeculae or cords of cells with scanty cytoplasm and finely granular chromatin positive for chromogranin (**f**), synaptophysin and other neuroendocrine markers

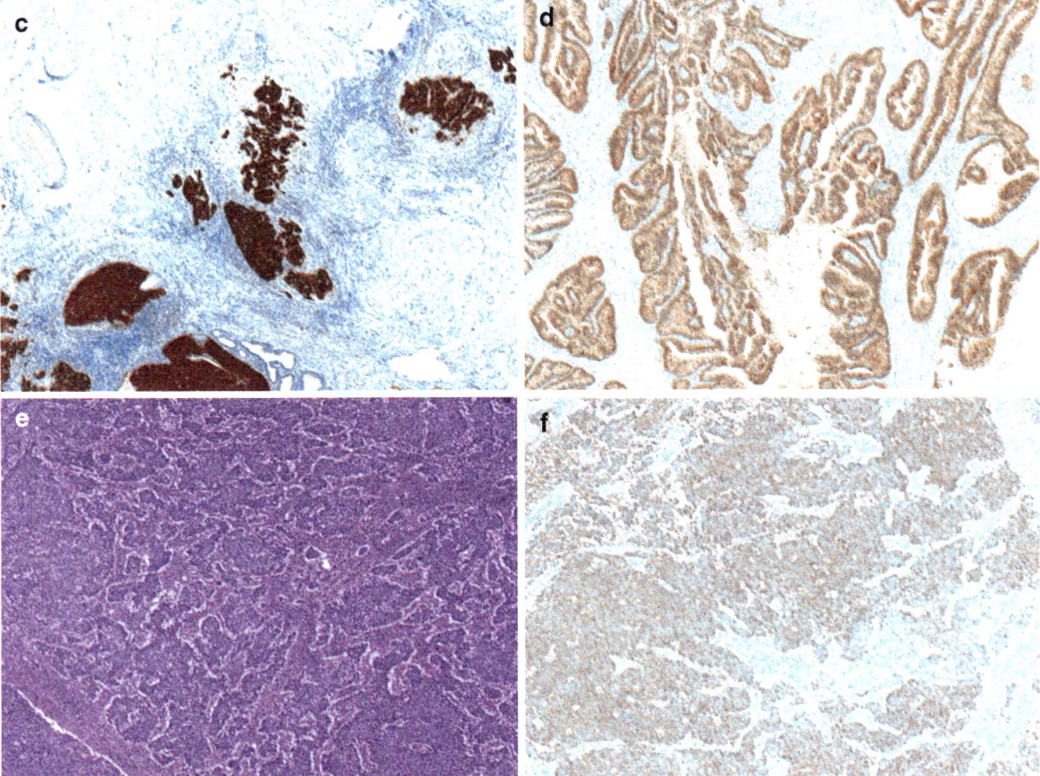

Fig. 3.2 (continued)

3.5 Staging

Staging of cervical cancer is defined according to the revised 2018 FIGO staging system (Fig. 3.3). In particular, stage IB is now divided into three subgroups: IB1 includes invasive tumour >5 mm and ≤2 cm in greatest diameter; IB2 includes tumours of 2–4 cm and IB3 includes tumours >4 cm.

The nodal involvement is now designed as stage IIIC and is divided into two subgroups: IIIC1 for pelvic lymph nodes (LNs) only and IIIC2 for para-aortic node involvement.

The revised 2018 FIGO staging system did not include the lymphovascular space invasion (LVSI). Early-stage cervical cancer concerns 2018 FIGO stages IA, IB1 and IB2 disease, whereas locally advanced cervical cancer (LACC) refers to 2018 FIGO stages IB3 to IVA disease [7].

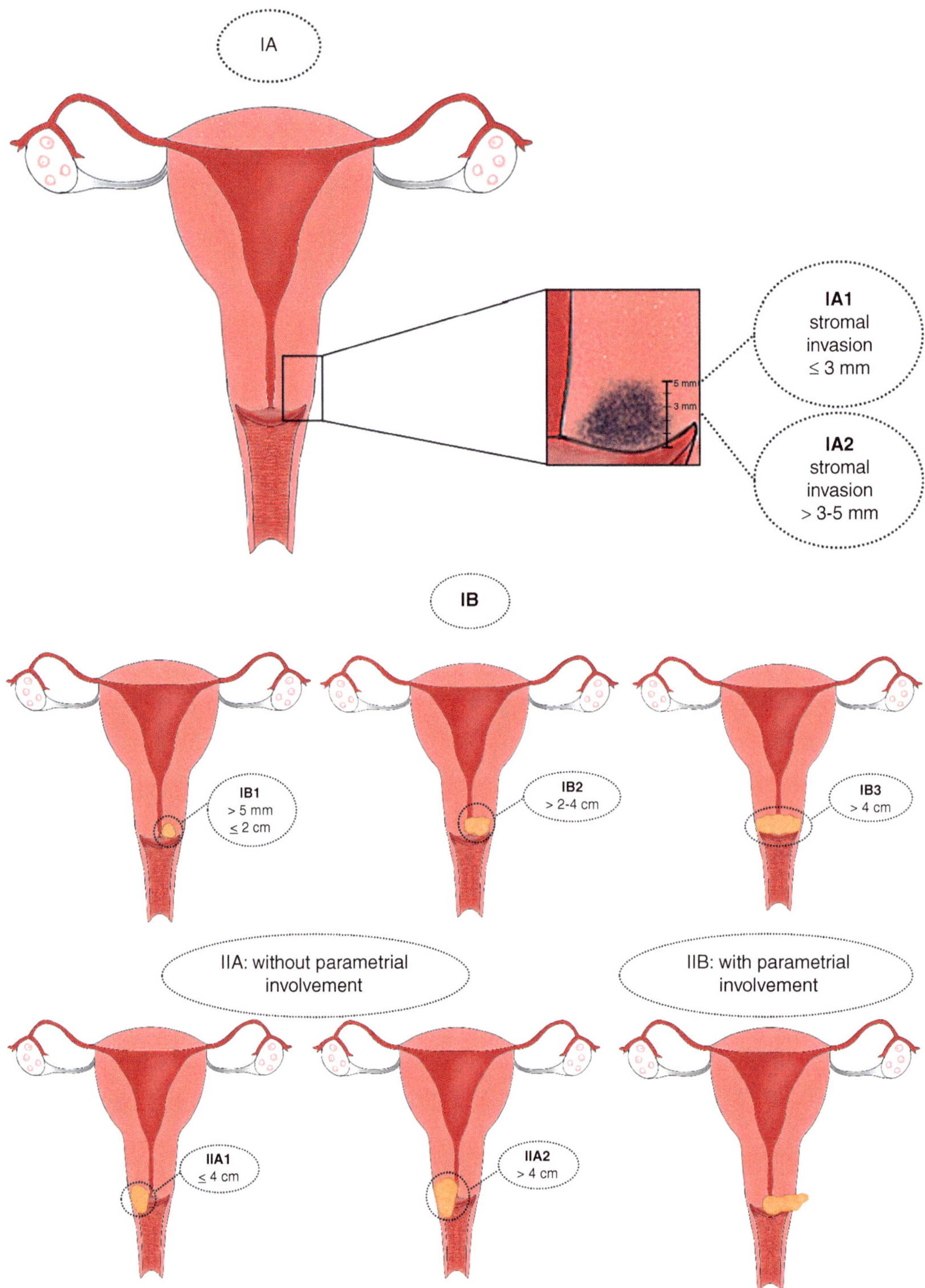

Fig. 3.3 2018 FIGO stages

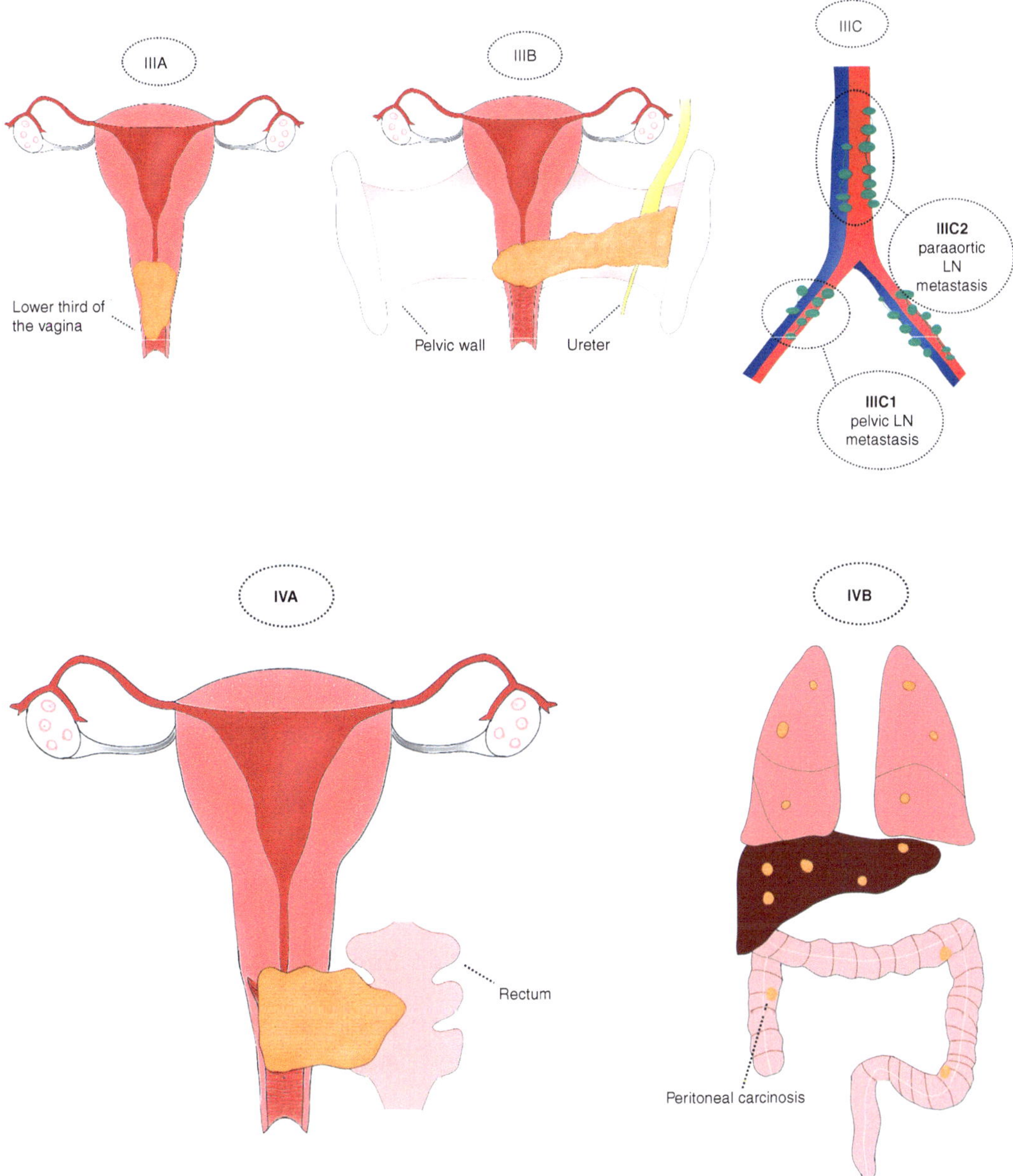

Fig. 3.3 (continued)

3.6 Lymphatic Drainage of the Cervix

The lymphatic drainage is bilateral because of the midline position of the uterine cervix. It is principally to the pelvic nodes (parametrial, internal iliac, external iliac and presacral nodes) and then to the common iliac and to the para-aortic nodes (Fig. 3.4) [8].

3.7 Sentinel Node Biopsy Versus Lymphadenectomy

The presence of nodal involvement is the most important prognostic factor in cervical cancer patients. The risk of pelvic lymph node (LN) involvement is low (21%) in early-stage disease, thus extensive pelvic LN dissection is considered an overtreatment with a high risk of post-operative complications (i.e. vessel and nerve injuries, ureteral wound, infections, lymphocele and lymphoedema).

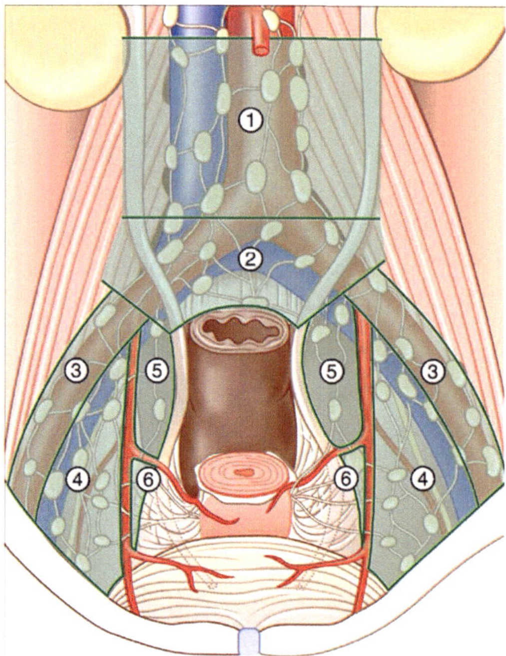

Fig. 3.4 Schematic representation of lymphatic drainage areas. 1: para-aortic area; 2: common iliac area; 3: external iliac area; 4: interiliac area; 5: internal iliac area and 6: parametrium area. Courtesy of Marnitz S, Köhler C, Bongardt S, Braig U, Hertel H, Schneider A. Topographic distribution of sentinel lymph nodes in patients with cervical cancer. Gynecol Oncol. 2006;103:35–44

Prospective and retrospective studies support the feasibility of sentinel node biopsy (SNB) in early-stage disease and suggest that extensive pelvic LN dissection may be safely avoided in selected patients.

SNB enables to identify unexpected lymphatic drainage patterns (i.e. parametrium, internal iliac, common iliac and para-aortic areas; Fig. 3.4, areas 6, 5, 2, 1) in early cervical cancer. In particular, the SENTICOL longitudinal study revealed that 13% (3/23) of patients with SN metastases had a single nodal metastasis in an unexpected area. Moreover, this study demonstrated that bilateral SNB provides a more reliable assessment of nodal involvement and leads to fewer false negatives than unilateral SNB.

The pathological evaluation of SNs with ultrastaging and immunohistochemistry results in an increased identification of micro-metastases (>0.2 and ≤2 mm in diameter) and isolated tumour cells (cells or cell clusters ≤0.2 mm in diameter), improving nodal staging. SNB should be done only in Centres with expertise and training [9–13].

3.8 Sentinel Node Mapping

3.8.1 Indications and Contraindications

Indications and contraindications of SN mapping are summarized in Table 3.1. If there is no mapping on a hemi-pelvis, a side-specific pelvic lymphadenectomy should be performed because the histological status of SNs in a hemi-pelvis does not predict the histology of contralateral nodes [14, 15].

3.8.2 Radiopharmaceuticals

The radiopharmaceuticals for SN mapping are colloids labelled with technetium-99m (^{99m}Tc) and are summarized in Table 3.2 [16, 17].

Table 3.1 Indications and contraindications for SN mapping

Indications	Contraindications
Clinically negative node (cN0) – IA1 (stromal invasion ≤3 mm in depth with lymphovascular space invasion) – IA2 (stromal invasion >3 mm and ≤5 mm in depth) – IB1 (invasive carcinoma >5 mm in depth of stromal invasion and ≤2 cm in greatest dimension) – IB2 (invasive carcinoma >2 cm and ≤4 cm in greatest dimension)	– Previous pelvic lymphadenectomy – Previous radiotherapy to pelvic nodes – Nodal involvement (N+) – Parametrial invasion

Table 3.2 Radiopharmaceuticals for SN mapping

Radiopharmaceuticals	Country	Particle size (nm)	Pros	Cons
^{99m}Tc-nanocolloid	Europe	5–80	Preoperative mapping	Radiation burden Preoperative injection
^{99m}Tc-sulphur colloid	United States	100–200 (filtered)		
^{99m}Tc-antimony trisulphide	Canada/ Australia	3–30		
Indocyanine green (ICG)-^{99m}Tc-nanocolloid	Europe	5–80	Preoperative and intraoperative mapping	

3.8.3 Administered Activity and Injection Sites

The radiopharmaceutical is injected into the cervix, usually at 2 or 4 points (Fig. 3.5) using a 20- or 22-gauge spinal needle and speculum (Fig. 3.6a).

The most frequently administered activity is about 110 MBq in four aliquots of 0.5 mL (total volume of 2 mL) in a 1-day protocol, while four aliquots of 220 MBq in 1 mL (total volume of 4 mL) are used in a 2-day protocol.

After cervical injection, the most common locations of pelvic SNs are medial to the external iliac vessels, ventral to the hypogastric vessels and in the superior part of the obturator space. The less frequent locations are in the common iliac and presacral area [14, 16].

3.8.4 Acquisition Protocol

Early (Fig. 3.6b) and late (Fig. 3.6c) planar images are acquired, respectively, at 30 and 120 min after radiotracer injection for 3–5 min in anterior and lateral views.

After acquisition of late planar images, single photon emission computed tomography/computed tomography (SPECT/CT) images are obtained (Fig. 3.6d) [16].

3.8.5 Pitfalls in Interpretation

Possible pitfalls are the false-positive SNs due to the retrograde radioactive leakage during the cervical injection in the vagina (radioactive contamination) or when the SN is metastatic, causing lymphatic stasis and bypass of lymphatic flow to other LNs. The false-positive SNs due to the radioactive contamination appear as a hot spot that can be easily detected with SPECT/CT while the hot spots due to metastatic nodes can be avoided with careful preoperative imaging that rules out gross nodal involvement.

Another possible pitfall can be the nonvisualization of SNs due to a deep injection, loss of injection fluid, overweight women or lymphatic stasis [18].

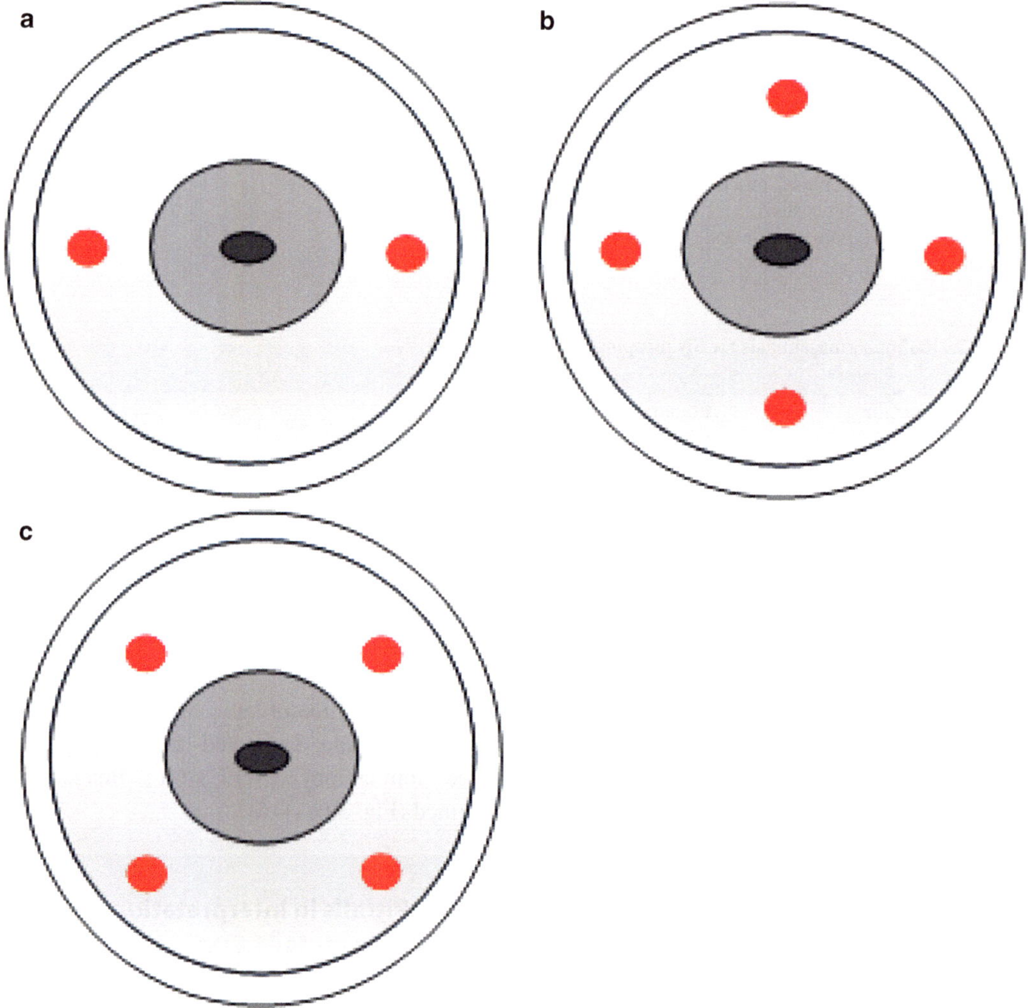

Fig. 3.5 Cervical injection at 2 (**a**) and 4 (**b**, **c**) points

3.8.6 Utility of SPECT/CT

Preoperative SPECT/CT provides three-dimensional images with better contrast and spatial resolution than planar images, resulting in precise anatomic localization of the SNs and depiction of additional SNs.

Moreover, SPECT/CT images are useful in the detection of SNs close to the injection site, as parametrial nodes, and SNs localized in uncommon locations, as para-aortic (Fig. 3.6d) and presacral nodes.

SPECT/CT helps in the visualization of bilateral drainage and reduces the false-positive SNs owing to the presence of radioactivity in enlarged lymphatic vessels [19–22].

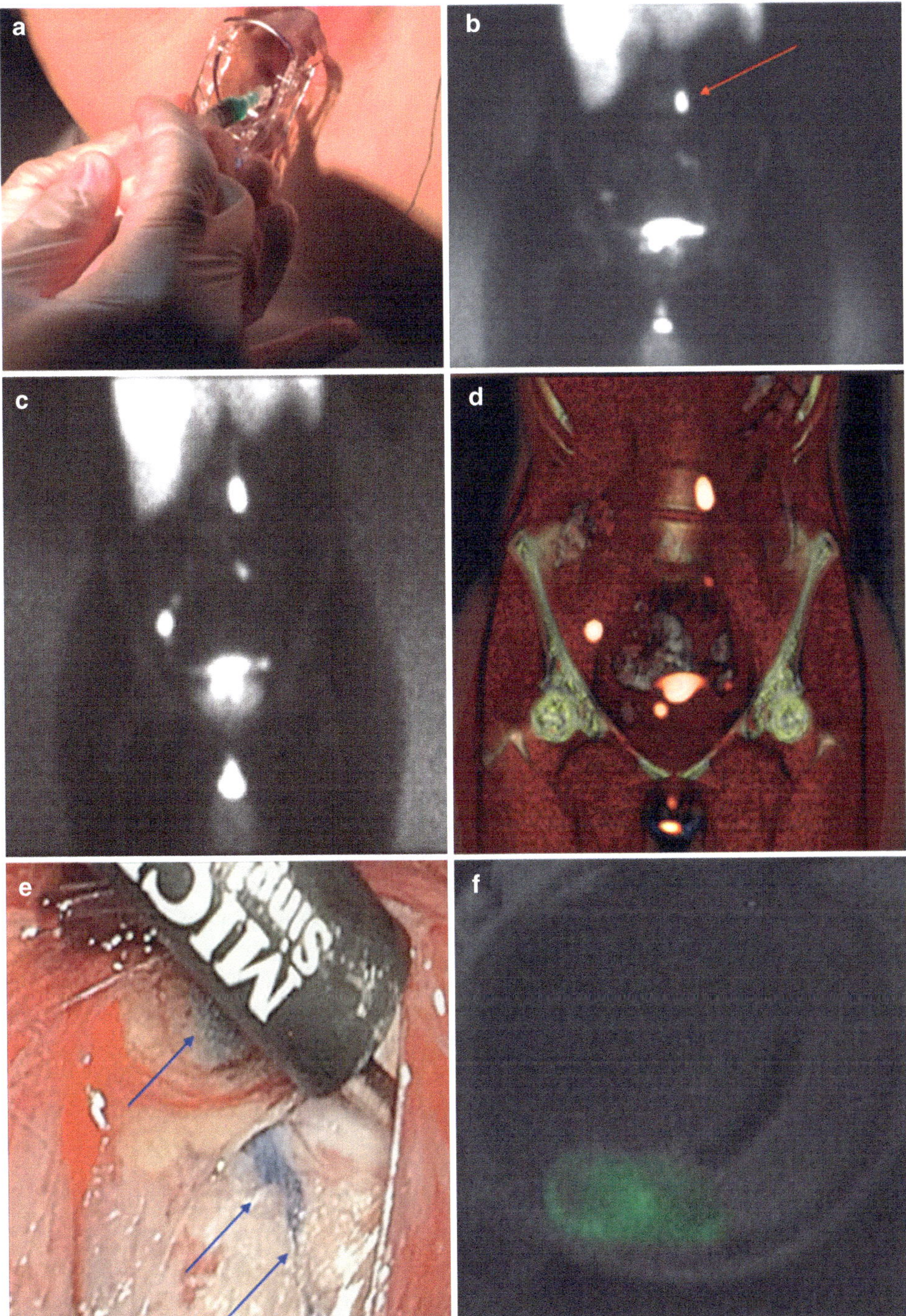

Fig. 3.6 SN mapping in cervical cancer. Cervical injection of ICG-^{99m}Tc-nanocolloid (**a**), early planar image (**b**) and late planar image (**c**) showing a para-aortic SN (red arrow). Coronal CT image with 3D volume rendering (**d**) showing the para-aortic SN with the surrounding anatomical structures. During laparoscopy (**e**) the para-aortic SN showing blue-stained lymphatic channel (blue arrows). The excised para-aortic SN was also fluorescent (**f**). Courtesy of Collarino A, Zurru A, Vidal-Sicart S. Preoperative and Intraoperative Lymphatic Mapping for Radioguided Sentinel Node Biopsy in Cancers of the Female Reproductive System. In: Mariani G, Vidal-Sicart S, Valdés Olmos R. Atlas of Lymphoscintigraphy and Sentinel Node Mapping. Springer, Cham. 2020. https://doi.org/10.1007/978-3-030-45296-4_14

3.9 Intraoperative Sentinel Node and Pathological Evaluation

Prior to surgery, an optical tracer, blue dye or ICG, is injected in the same points as the radiotracer injection (total volume of 2–4 mL). In some Centres, mainly in the United States, the optical tracer is the one method applied. If the radiopharmaceutical is injected (intraoperative counting), a laparoscopic gamma probe is used during laparoscopic surgery.

When available, a portable gamma camera could be particularly useful, allowing a better localization of parametrial SNs, as well as a better discrimination of para-aortic SNs from physiologic liver activity, and assessment of completeness of SNs excision in the surgical bed. A fluorescence probe must be used if ICG is injected. After excision of SNs, ex vivo radioactivity of SNs (ex vivo counting) and/or the near-infrared rays of fluorescent SNs are measured (Fig. 3.6f).

All excised SNs are sent for haematoxylin and eosin (H&E) staining. If the H&E staining of SNs does not reveal metastases, ultra-staging should be performed to rule out micro-metastatic disease. Metastatic SNs guide for a more extensive lymphadenectomy or for adjuvant therapy [23].

3.10 PET/CT and Cervical Cancer

3.10.1 Indications and Contraindications

For clinical routine, ^{18}F-fluorodeoxyglucose (^{18}F-FDG) is used. Indications and contraindications of ^{18}F-FDG positron emission tomography/computed tomography (PET/CT) are summarized in Table 3.3.

In patients with neuroendocrine cervical carcinoma (more frequently, small cell type), PET/CT imaging using ^{68}Ga-labelled somatostatin analogue peptides may be useful to assess the expression of somatostatin receptors by tumour lesions [5, 14, 24].

Table 3.3 Indications and contraindications for ^{18}F-FDG PET/CT in cervical cancer

Indications	Contraindications
Staging – In women with FIGO stage ≥IB1 to evaluate nodal and distant disease Response assessment – In women with FIGO stage IB3 to IVA disease Suspected local or distant recurrence Follow-up/surveillance – In women with FIGO stage IB3 at 3–6 months after treatment – In women with FIGO stage II-IVA within 3–6 months after therapy – In stage IVB to assess response or to define further therapy	Glucose blood level > 200 mg/dl Pregnancy

3.10.2 Acquisition Protocol

The patient should fast for 6 h before the exam and should have a glucose blood level lower than 200 mg/dl. ^{18}F-FDG is intravenously injected and the patient is hydrated with 500 ml of saline solution to ensure a low concentration of ^{18}F-FDG in the urine. The intravenous furosemide injection is helpful for flushing out excreted ^{18}F-FDG, avoiding urinary artefacts in case of suspected recurrence on the vaginal vault. Low-dose CT scan is acquired from the skull to the pelvis for anatomical localization and attenuation correction. PET/CT images are acquired at 60 min (±10 min) after ^{18}F-FDG injection in the range defined by CT [25].

3.10.3 Image Analysis

For visual analysis, any focus of ^{18}F-FDG uptake at the primary site and at the LN sites and/or distant sites higher than the surrounding background is considered abnormal and interpreted as positive.

For quantitative analysis, maximum standardized uptake value (SUV_{max}) is the most widely used quantitative parameter. SUV_{max} is defined as the hottest voxel within the volume of interest (VOI).

SUV_{max}	19.2
SUV_{peak}	10.45/size 1cm^3
SUV_{mean}	10.4
MTV	3.3 cm^3
TLG	34.5
Threshold	7.69/40%

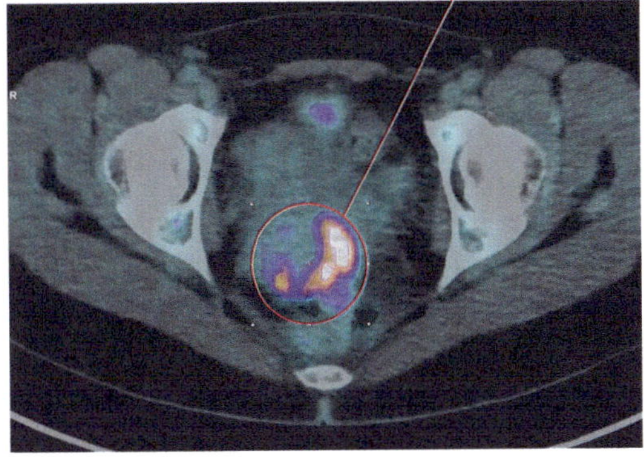

Fig. 3.7 Quantitative parameters

Also, SUV_{peak} (mean SUV of a sphere of 12-mm diameter centred on SUV_{max}) and SUV_{mean} (mean SUV within the tumour) are frequently used.

Volumetric PET parameters are metabolic tumour volume (MTV), which represents the volume of functioning cells, and total lesion glycolysis (TLG = MTV x SUV_{mean}), which combines the metabolic and volumetric information of the entire tumour (Fig. 3.7).

3.10.4 Pitfalls in Interpretation

Possible pitfalls in interpretation are due to physiological ^{18}F-FDG uptake within the endometrial cavity and the ovaries (Fig. 3.8a) during the menstrual and ovulatory phases as well as within benign fibroids or endometriotic cysts. The phys-

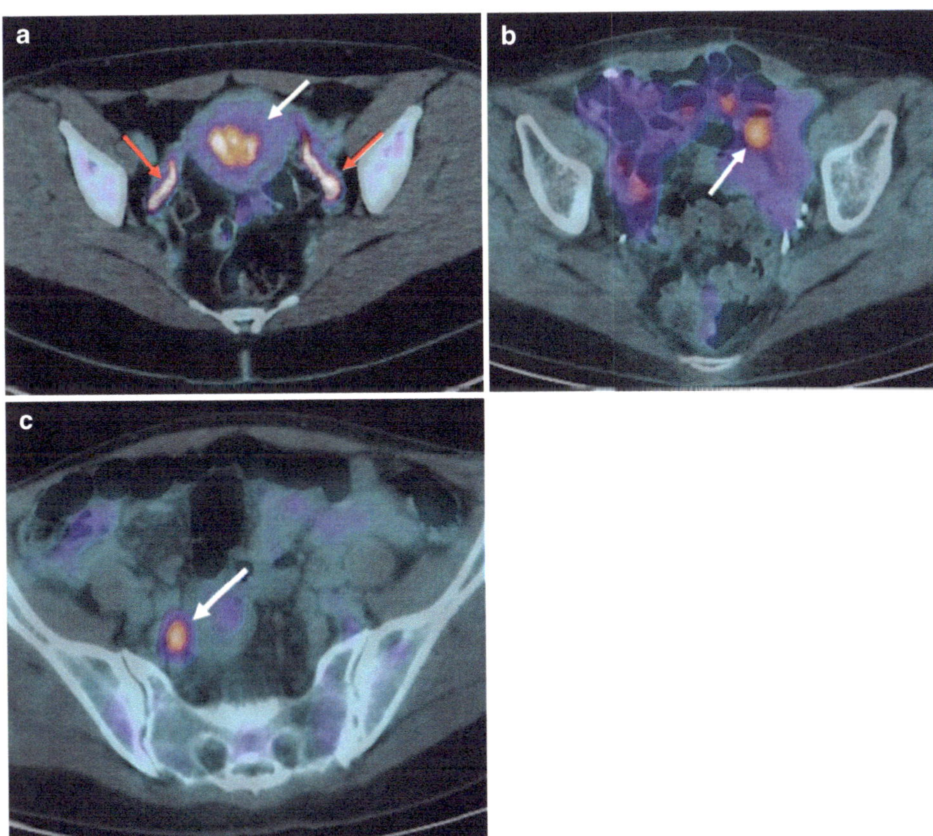

Fig. 3.8 Transverse fused PET/CT image (**a**) shows focal physiological endometrial uptake (white arrow) and physiological adnexal uptake (red arrows). Transverse fused PET/CT image (**b**) shows a focal uptake corresponding to the physiological bowel activity (white arrow). Transverse fused PET/CT image (**c**) shows a focal uptake corresponding to the ureteral urinary activity (white arrow)

iological bowel activity (Fig. 3.8b), when focal, and focal ureteric (Fig. 3.8c) or bladder activity can be mistaken for pathological uptake in the pelvis.

False-negative results are usually due to small primary tumours (FIGO IA, <1 cm) or small (<5 mm) LNs or peritoneal diseases that are below the resolution of PET/CT, as well as necrotic LNs (Fig. 3.9) [26].

3.11 Diagnostic Utility of PET/CT

3.11.1 Staging and Therapy Planning

Cervical tumours are usually highly ^{18}F-FDG avid, with higher values of tracer uptake for SCC than mucinous adenocarcinoma (Fig. 3.10).

According to international guidelines, PET/CT is recommended for staging LACC (stage IB3 to

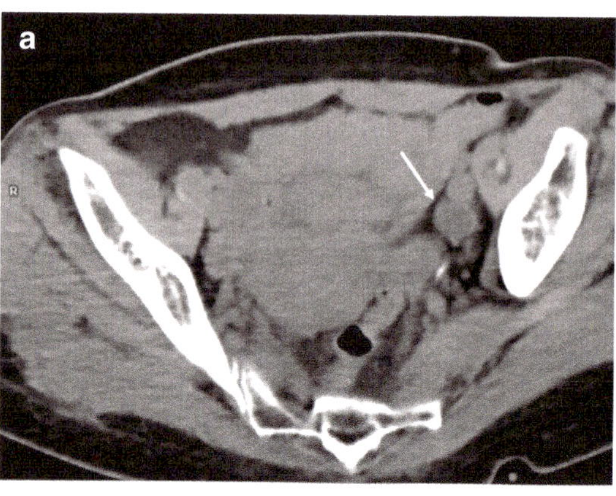

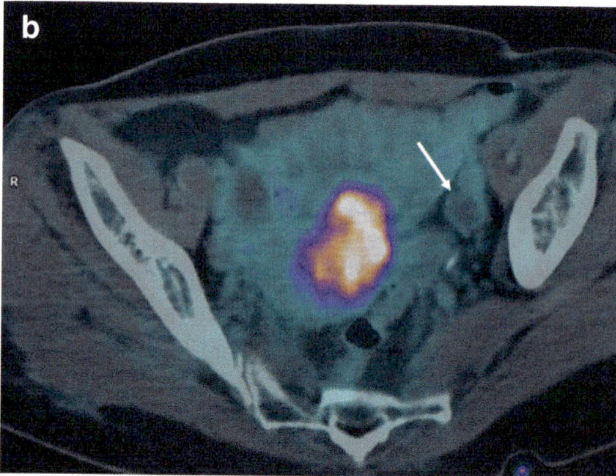

Fig. 3.9 A 56-year-old woman with squamous cell carcinoma of uterine cervix. Transverse low-dose CT image (**a**) shows one left obturator lymph node with short axis of 11 mm, round shape, necrosis (arrow) and without uptake on transverse fused PET/CT image (**b**, arrow)

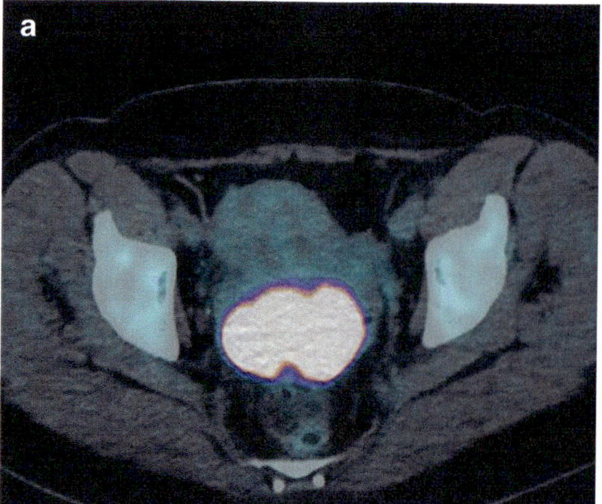

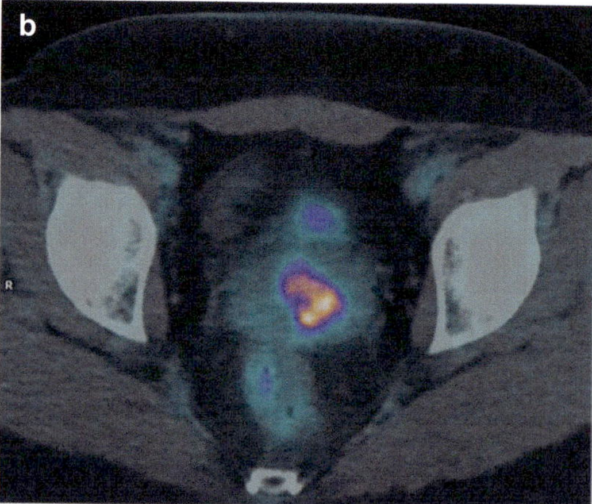

Fig. 3.10 Transverse fused PET/CT image (**a**) shows a high and homogenous ^{18}F-FDG uptake (SUV_{max} 36.49) corresponding to a squamous cell carcinoma of uterine cervix. Transverse fused PET/CT image (**b**) shows an inhomogeneous ^{18}F-FDG uptake (SUV_{max} 11.80) corresponding to adenocarcinoma of uterine cervix

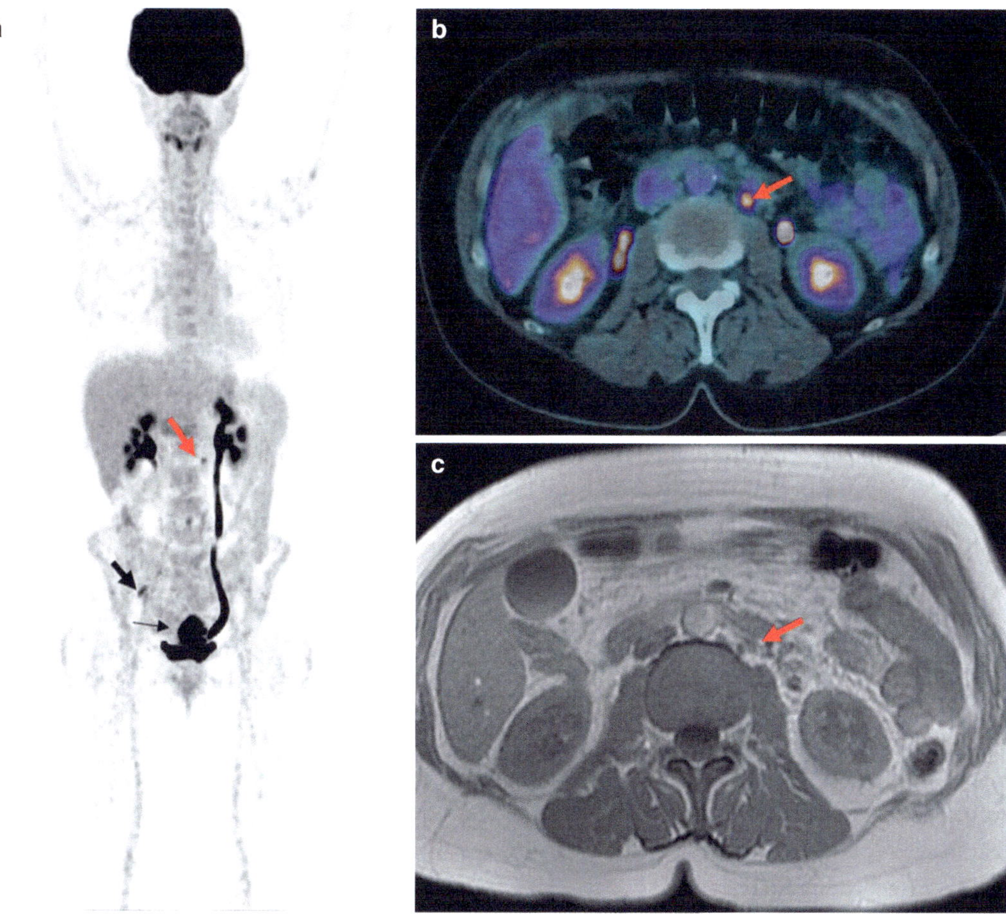

Fig. 3.11 A 61-year-old woman with squamous cell carcinoma of the uterine cervix. Multiple intensity projection images (**a**) show ^{18}F-FDG uptake of the primary tumour (T, thin black arrow), one right obturator lymph node (thick black arrow) and one left para-aortic lymph node (red arrow). Transverse fused PET/CT image (**b**) shows a focal ^{18}F-FDG uptake in one left para-aortic lymph node (red arrow, short axis of 5 mm and SUV_{max} 5.5) not suspicious on transverse T1 weighted magnetic resonance image (**c**, red arrow)

IVA disease), in particular LN and distant metastases (Fig. 3.11), as primary tumour extent (T-staging) is carried out with magnetic resonance (MR). In early-stage disease, PET/CT has a low sensitivity (32.1%) in detecting nodal disease because of the low prevalence of nodal involvement and the presence of micro-metastases (<5 mm, below the PET/CT resolution).

In LACC, the prevalence of pelvic nodal involvement is high, varying from 15% to 65%. PET/CT has a high pooled sensitivity (0.88, 95%CI: 0.40–0.99) and pooled specificity (0.93, 95%CI: 0.85–0.97) for detecting pelvic nodal disease. Interestingly, only 73% of patients with enlarged pelvic LNs at MR are PET positive; however, only 5% of recurrences are found in patients with enlarged LNs and negative PET. Therefore, in these patients a negative PET is a favourable prognostic factor. According to international guidelines, pelvic nodes are always included in the radiation therapy field.

In patients with positive PET at pelvic LN level, additional treatment or boosting of the pelvic LNs as well as a close follow-up to monitor for disease recurrence are indicated. In LACC, the detection of para-aortic lymph node (PALN) disease is crucial to extent of the radiation therapy field. Patients with positive PET at PALN level receive a treatment modification with extension of RT field to T12-L1 level.

Although the prevalence of PALN involvement is high (15–70%), PET/CT has a low pooled sensitivity (0.40, 95%CI: 0.18–0.66) for detecting PALN disease. False-negative (FN) results are mainly due to PALNs with micro-metastases (≤5 mm), hence below the PET/CT resolution. According to ESGO guidelines, laparoscopic PALN dissection may be considered in patients with negative PALN on pretreatment PET/CT for staging purposes. It is unclear if patients' survival could benefit from laparoscopic surgical PALN staging before chemoradiotherapy. A prospective multicentre study investigated the therapeutic impact on survival of laparoscopic PA staging in 237 LACC patients with negative PET of the para-aortic area. The PALN involvement was 12%. In any case, the survival rate of patients with PALN metastases ≤5 mm was similar to that of patients without PALN metastases.

False-positive results are due to ^{18}F-FDG uptake by inflammatory nodes or to misinterpretation of physiological uptake. The pooled specificity of PET/CT for detecting para-aortic disease is high (0.93, 95%CI: 0.91–0.95). When both pelvic and PA nodes are PET positive, the surgical PA staging is omitted and the radiation therapy field is extended to PA nodes.

Regarding distant metastases, PET/CT has a high specificity (97.7%) for detecting distant metastases (i.e. lung, omentum, bone and liver).

Combined or integrated PET and MR could be an important tool in the staging of cervical cancer by assessing the primary tumour with MR and evaluating nodal and distant disease with PET. Moreover, digital PET scanners with higher spatial resolution may improve the diagnostic performance of PET/CT for detecting small LNs and distant metastases [27–31].

3.11.2 Prognostic Stratification

High SUV_{max} of the primary tumour is predictive of an increased risk of LN metastasis at diagnosis, persistent disease after chemoradiotherapy (CRT), pelvic recurrence and worse survival. High TLG of primary tumour is predictive of relapse and death. High SUV_{max} of pelvic LN is predictive of persistent pelvic disease after CRT, pelvic recurrence and worse disease-specific survival. High SUV_{max} of PALN is predictive of recurrence and death in patients with cervical cancer [32–35].

3.11.3 Response Assessment

In LACC patients, ^{18}F-FDG PET/CT performed at baseline and at 3 months post completion of therapy is routinely used for response assessment. Baseline (pretreatment) PET/CT helps to tailor treatment, while post-therapy PET/CT is useful to assess metabolic response (Figs. 3.12 and 3.13) and to predict prognosis.

In particular, complete metabolic response (CMR) on post-therapy has a lower failure rate and higher overall survival rate compared to partial metabolic response (PMR)/progressive disease (PD).

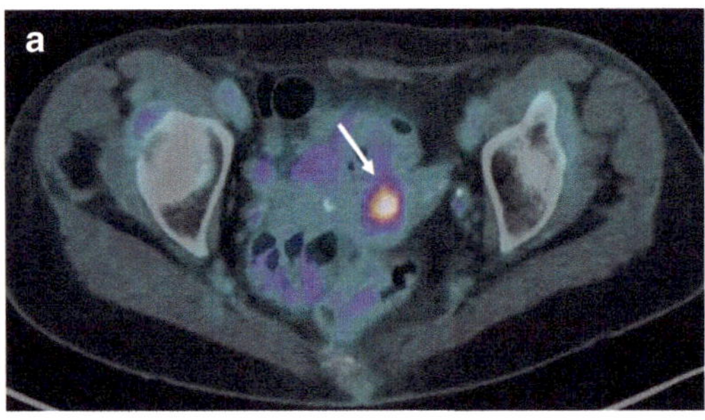

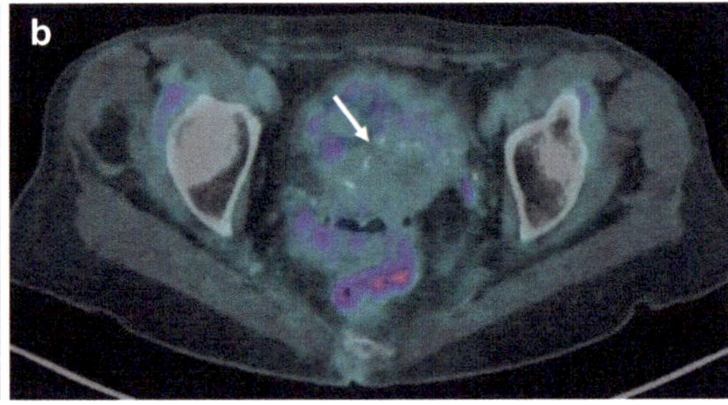

Fig. 3.12 A 81-year-old woman with cervical cancer. Transverse fused PET/CT images show an intense focal uptake corresponding to a squamous cell carcinoma of the uterine cervix (white arrow) prior to chemoradiotherapy (**a**) and no uptake (white arrow) after therapy (**b**), indicative of complete metabolic response

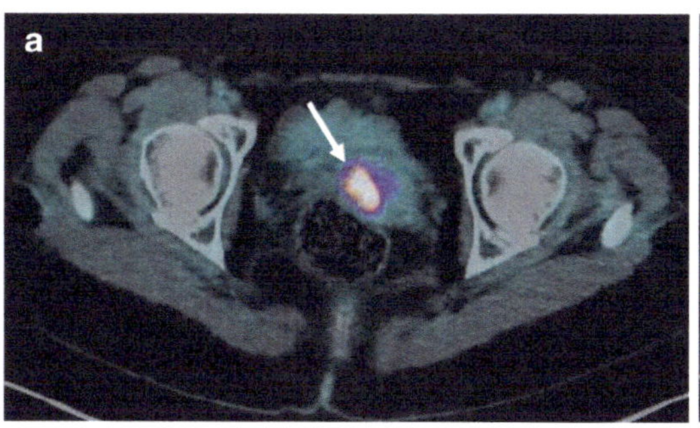

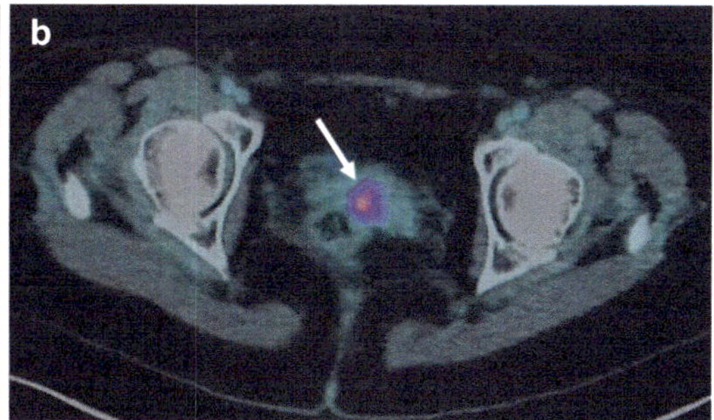

Fig. 3.13 A 52-year-old woman with cervical cancer. Transverse fused PET/CT images show an intense focal uptake (white arrow) corresponding to a squamous cell carcinoma of the uterine cervix prior to chemoradiotherapy (**a**) and a mild uptake (white arrow) after therapy (**b**), indicative of partial metabolic response

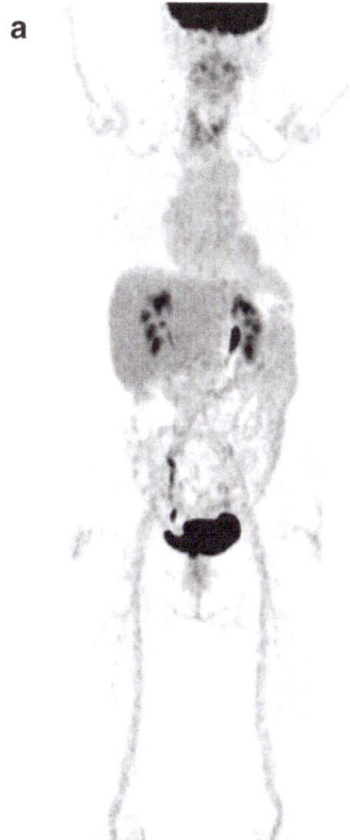

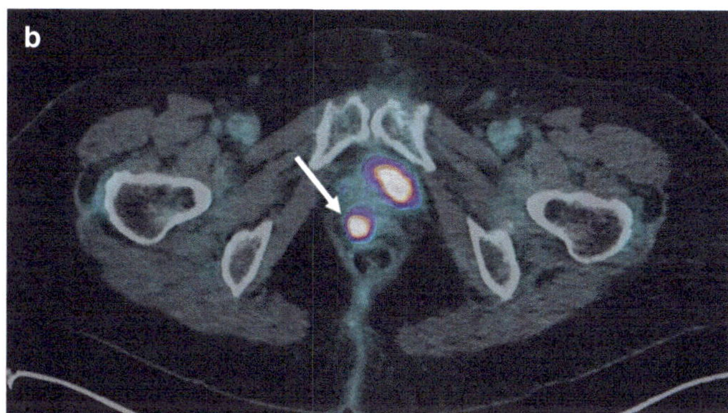

Fig. 3.14 An 81-year-old woman with squamous cell carcinoma of the uterine cervix underwent a restaging PET/CT (**a**, multiple intensity projection images) for suspected pelvic recurrence. Transverse fused PET/CT image (**b**) shows a focal ^{18}F-FDG uptake on the vaginal vault (white arrow)

In addition, post-therapy PET/CT has a higher negative predictive value (NPV) than positive predictive value (PPV) due to the high false-positive rate in the PMR group. PET/CT performed early during CRT could identify a subgroup with CMR who has an excellent prognosis. However, early PET/CT has a limited utility for response prediction due to the low PPV in PMR patients [36–38].

3.11.4 Restaging for Suspected Recurrence

Disease recurrence occurs in approximately one-third of patients with LACC within the first 2 years after therapy. The sites of recurrence are vaginal vault (Fig. 3.14), parametrial and pelvic wall, PALN and supraclavicular LNs, and distant metastases including peritoneal disease.

The survival rate after recurrence is low and the cure efficacy is minimal. Therefore, the early detection of recurrence could improve the survival of these patients.

MR and CT are limited in identifying LN metastases and extra pelvic metastases after therapy because of the difficulty in differentiating disease from scarring or inflammation caused by therapy.

In case of suspected recurrence, PET/CT had a higher sensitivity (92%) in detection of nodal and extra pelvic relapse compared to CT and MR [39–41].

References

1. Bray F, Ferlay J, Soerjomataram I, Siegel RL, Torre LA, Jemal A. Global cancer statistics 2018: GLOBOCAN estimates of incidence and mortality worldwide for 36 cancers in 185 countries. CA Cancer J Clin. 2018;68(6):394–424. https://doi.org/10.3322/caac.21492.
2. SEER Cancer Stat Facts: Cervical Cancer. National Cancer Institute, Bethesda. https://seer.cancer.gov/statfacts/html/cervix.html. Accessed Dec 2021.
3. Dugué PA, Rebolj M, Garred P, Lynge E. Immunosuppression and risk of cervical cancer. Expert Rev Anticancer Ther. 2013;13(1):29–42. https://doi.org/10.1586/era.12.159.
4. Kjær SK, Frederiksen K, Munk C, Iftner T. Long-term absolute risk of cervical intraepithelial neoplasia grade 3 or worse following human papillomavirus infection: role of persistence. J Natl Cancer Inst. 2010;102(19):1478–88. https://doi.org/10.1093/jnci/djq356.
5. Inzani F, Santoro A, Angelico G, Feraco A, Spadola S, Arciuolo D, et al. Neuroendocrine carcinoma of the uterine cervix: a clinicopathologic and immunohistochemical study with focus on novel markers (Sst2–Sst5). Cancers (Basel). 2020;12(5):1211. https://doi.org/10.3390/cancers12051211.
6. WHO classification of Tumours Editorial Board. Female genital tumours. In: WHO classification of tumours. 5th ed. Lyon: International Agency for Research on Cancer; 2020.
7. Bhatla N, Berek JS, Cuello Fredes M, Denny LA, Grenman S, Karunaratne K, et al. Revised FIGO staging for carcinoma of the cervix uteri. Int J Gynaecol Obstet. 2019;145:129–35. https://doi.org/10.1002/ijgo.12749.
8. Benedetti-Panici P, Maneschi F, Scambia G, Greggi S, Cutillo G, D'Andrea G, et al. Lymphatic spread of cervical cancer: an anatomical and pathological study based on 225 radical hysterectomies with systematic pelvic and aortic lymphadenectomy. Gynecol Oncol. 1996;62(1):19–24. https://doi.org/10.1006/gyno.1996.0184.
9. Altgassen C, Hertel H, Brandstädt A, Köhler C, Dürst M, Schneider A. Multicenter validation study of the sentinel lymph node concept in cervical cancer: AGO study group. J Clin Oncol. 2008;26(18):2943–51. https://doi.org/10.1200/JCO.2007.13.8933.
10. Bats AS, Frati A, Mathevet P, Orliaguet I, Querleu D, Zerdoud S, et al. Contribution of lymphoscintigraphy to intraoperative sentinel lymph node detection in early cervical cancer: analysis of the prospective multicenter SENTICOL cohort. Gynecol Oncol. 2015;137(2):264–9. https://doi.org/10.1016/j.ygyno.2015.02.018.
11. Bats AS, Mathevet P, Buenerd A, Orliaguet I, Mery E, Zerdoud S, et al. The sentinel node technique detects unexpected drainage pathways and allows nodal ultrastaging in early cervical cancer: insights from the multicenter prospective SENTICOL study. Ann Surg Oncol. 2013 Feb;20(2):413–22. https://doi.org/10.1245/s10434-012-2597-7.
12. Cibula D, Abu-Rustum NR, Dusek L, Slama J, Zikán M, Zaal A, et al. Bilateral ultrastaging of sentinel lymph node in cervical cancer: lowering the false-negative rate and improving the detection of micrometastasis. Gynecol Oncol. 2012 Dec;127(3):462–6. https://doi.org/10.1016/j.ygyno.2012.08.035.
13. Lécuru F, Mathevet P, Querleu D, Leblanc E, Morice P, Daraï E, et al. Bilateral negative sentinel nodes accurately predict absence of lymph node metastasis in early cervical cancer: results of the SENTICOL study. J Clin Oncol. 2011;29(13):1686–91. https://doi.org/10.1200/JCO.2010.32.0432.
14. Abu-Rustum NR, Yashar CM, Bradley K, Brooks R, Campos SM, Chino J, et al. Cervical Cancer: version 1.2022. In: NCCN Clinical Practice Guidelines in Oncology (NCCN guidelines); 2021. https://www.nccn.org/professionals/physician_gls/pdf/cervical.pdf. Accessed 12 Dec 2021.
15. Cormier B, Diaz JP, Shih K, Sampson RM, Sonoda Y, Park KJ, et al. Establishing a sentinel lymph node mapping algorithm for the treatment of early cervical cancer. Gynecol Oncol. 2011;122(2):275–80. https://doi.org/10.1016/j.ygyno.2011.04.023.
16. Giammarile F, Bozkurt MF, Cibula D, Pahisa J, Oyen WJ, Paredes P, et al. The EANM clinical and technical guidelines for lymphoscintigraphy and sentinel node localization in gynaecological cancers. Eur J Nucl Med Mol Imaging. 2014;41:1463–77. https://doi.org/10.1007/s00259-014-2732-8.
17. Paredes P, Vidal-Sicart S, Campos F, Tapias A, Sánchez N, Martínez S, et al. Role of ICG-99mTc-nanocolloid for sentinel lymph node detection in cervical cancer: a pilot study. Eur J Nucl Med Mol Imaging. 2017;44(11):1853–61. https://doi.org/10.1007/s00259-017-3706-4.
18. Collarino A, Zurru A, Vidal-Sicart S. Preoperative and intraoperative lymphatic mapping for Radioguided

sentinel node biopsy in cancers of the female reproductive system. In: Mariani G, Vidal-Sicart S, Valdés Olmos R, editors. Atlas of lymphoscintigraphy and sentinel node mapping. Cham: Springer; 2020. https://doi.org/10.1007/978-3-030-45296-4_14.
19. Belhocine TZ, Prefontaine M, Lanvin D, Bertrand M, Rachinsky I, Ettler H, et al. Added-value of SPECT/CT to lymphatic mapping and sentinel lymphadenectomy in gynaecological cancers. Am J Nucl Med Mol Imaging. 2013;3(2):182–93.
20. Kraft O, Havel M. Detection of sentinel lymph nodes in gynecologic tumours by planar scintigraphy and SPECT/CT. Mol Imaging Radionucl Ther. 2012;21(2):47–55. https://doi.org/10.4274/Mirt.236.
21. Martínez A, Zerdoud S, Mery E, Bouissou E, Ferron G, Querleu D. Hybrid imaging by SPECT/CT for sentinel lymph node detection in patients with cancer of the uterine cervix. Gynecol Oncol. 2010;119(3):431–5. https://doi.org/10.1016/j.ygyno.2010.08.001.
22. Pandit-Taskar N, Gemignani ML, Lyall A, Larson SM, Barakat RR, Abu Rustum NR. Single photon emission computed tomography SPECT-CT improves sentinel node detection and localization in cervical and uterine malignancy. Gynecol Oncol. 2010;117(1):59–64. https://doi.org/10.1016/j.ygyno.2009.12.021.
23. Collarino A, Vidal-Sicart S, Perotti G, Valdés Olmos RA. The sentinel node approach in gynaecological malignancies. Clin Transl Imaging. 2016;4:411–20. https://doi.org/10.1007/s40336-016-0187-6.
24. Damian A, Lago G, Rossi S, Alonso O, Engler H. Early detection of bone metastasis in small cell neuroendocrine carcinoma of the cervix by 68Ga-DOTATATE PET/CT imaging. Clin Nucl Med. 2017;42(3):216–7. https://doi.org/10.1097/RLU.0000000000001498.
25. Boellaard R, Delgado-Bolton R, Oyen WJG, Giammarile F, Tatsch K, Eschner W, et al. FDG PET/CT: EANM procedure guidelines for tumour imaging: version 2.0. Eur J Nucl Med Mol Imaging. 2015;42(2):328–54. https://doi.org/10.1007/s00259-014-2961-x.
26. Lakhani A, Khan SR, Bharwani N, Stewart V, Rockall AG, Khan S, et al. FDG PET/CT pitfalls in gynecologic and genitourinary oncologic imaging. Radiographics. 2017;37(2):577–94. https://doi.org/10.1148/rg.2017160059.
27. Adam JA, van Diepen PR, Mom CH, Stoker J, van Eck-Smit BLF, Bipat S. [18F]FDG-PET or PET/CT in the evaluation of pelvic and para-aortic lymph nodes in patients with locally advanced cervical cancer: a systematic review of the literature. Gynecol Oncol. 2020;159(2):588–96. https://doi.org/10.1016/j.ygyno.2020.08.021.
28. Gouy S, Morice P, Narducci F, Uzan C, Martinez A, Rey A, et al. Prospective multicenter study evaluating the survival of patients with locally advanced cervical cancer undergoing laparoscopic para-aortic lymphadenectomy before chemoradiotherapy in the era of positron emission tomography imaging. J Clin Oncol. 2013;31(24):3026–33. https://doi.org/10.1200/JCO.2012.47.3520.
29. Kidd EA, Spencer CR, Huettner PC, Siegel BA, Dehdashti F, Rader JS, et al. Cervical cancer histology and tumor differentiation affect 18F-fluorodeoxyglucose uptake. Cancer. 2009;115(15):3548–54. https://doi.org/10.1002/cncr.24400.
30. Lin A, Ma S, Dehdashti F, Markovina S, Schwarz J, Siegel B, et al. Detection of distant metastatic disease by positron emission tomography with 18 F-fluorodeoxyglucose (FDG-PET) at initial staging of cervical carcinoma. Int J Gynecol Cancer. 2019;29(3):487–91. https://doi.org/10.1136/ijgc-2018-000108.
31. Nguyen NC, Beriwal S, Moon CH, Furlan A, Mountz JM, Rangaswamy B. 18F-FDG PET/MRI primary staging of cervical Cancer: a pilot study with PET/CT comparison. J Nucl Med Technol. 2020;48(4):331–5. https://doi.org/10.2967/jnmt.120.247080.
32. Kidd EA, Siegel BA, Dehdashti F, Grigsby PW. The standardized uptake value for F-18 fluorodeoxyglucose is a sensitive predictive biomarker for cervical cancer treatment response and survival. Cancer. 2007;110(8):1738–44. https://doi.org/10.1002/cncr.22974.
33. Kidd EA, Siegel BA, Dehdashti F, Grigsby PW. Pelvic lymph node F-18 fluorodeoxyglucose uptake as a prognostic biomarker in newly diagnosed patients with locally advanced cervical cancer. Cancer. 2010;116(6):1469–75. https://doi.org/10.1002/cncr.24972.
34. Yen TC, See LC, Lai CH, Tsai CS, Chao A, Hsueh S, et al. Standardized uptake value in para-aortic lymph nodes is a significant prognostic factor in patients with primary advanced squamous cervical cancer. Eur J Nucl Med Mol Imaging. 2008;35(3):493–501. https://doi.org/10.1007/s00259-007-0612-1.
35. Yoo J, Choi JY, Moon SH, Bae DS, Bin PS, Choe YS, et al. Prognostic significance of volume-based metabolic parameters in uterine cervical cancer determined using 18F-fluorodeoxyglucose positron emission tomography. Int J Gynecol Cancer. 2012;22(7):1226–33. https://doi.org/10.1097/IGC.0b013e318260a905.
36. Lima GM, Matti A, Vara G, Dondi G, Naselli N, De Crescenzo EM, et al. Prognostic value of posttreatment 18F-FDG PET/CT and predictors of metabolic response to therapy in patients with locally advanced cervical cancer treated with concomitant chemoradiation therapy: an analysis of intensity- and volume-based PET parameters. Eur J Nucl Med Mol Imaging. 2018;45(12):2139–46. https://doi.org/10.1007/s00259-018-4077-1.
37. Kidd EA, Thomas M, Siegel BA, Dehdashti F, Grigsby PW. Changes in cervical cancer FDG uptake during chemoradiation and association with response. Int J Radiat Oncol Biol Phys. 2013;85(1):116–22. https://doi.org/10.1016/j.ijrobp.2012.02.056.
38. Schwarz JK, Siegel BA, Dehdashti F, Grigsby PW. Metabolic response on post-therapy FDG-PET predicts patterns of failure after radiotherapy for cervical cancer. Int J Radiat Oncol Biol Phys. 2012;83(1):185–90. https://doi.org/10.1016/j.ijrobp.2011.05.053.
39. Chong GO, Lee WK, Jeong SY, Park SH, Lee YH, Lee SW, et al. Prognostic value of intratumoral metabolic

heterogeneity on F-18 fluorodeoxyglucose positron emission tomography/computed tomography in locally advanced cervical cancer patients treated with concurrent chemoradiotherapy. Oncotarget. 2017;8(52):90402–12. https://doi.org/10.18632/oncotarget.18769.

40. Grigsby PW, Siegel BA, Dehdashti F, Rader J, Zoberi I. Posttherapy [18F] fluorodeoxyglucose positron emission tomography in carcinoma of the cervix: response and outcome. J Clin Oncol. 2004;22(11):2167–71. doi: 10.1200/JCO.2004.09.035

41. Lai CH, Huang KG, See LC, Yen TC, Tsai CS, Chang TC, et al. Restaging of recurrent cervical carcinoma with dual-phase [18f]fluoro-2-deoxy-D-glucose positron emission tomography. Cancer. 2004;100(3):544–52. https://doi.org/10.1002/cncr.11928.

Endometrial Cancer

4

Pilar Paredes, Blanca Paño, Berta Díaz, and Sergi Vidal-Sicart

4.1 General Aspects

4.1.1 Anatomy and Lymphatic Drainage

4.1.1.1 Routes of Spreading of Disease

This tumor has a progressive locoregional spread, with a relatively low incidence of distant metastases. However, the distribution of metastatic sites is relatively at random. There are four routes of dissemination:

P. Paredes
Nuclear Medicine Department, Hospital Clínic Barcelona (CDI), Barcelona, Spain

Faculty of Medicine, University of Barcelona, Barcelona, Spain

Institut d'Investigacions Biomèdiques August Pi i Sunyer (IDIBAPS), Barcelona, Spain

B. Paño
Radiology Department, Hospital Clínic de Barcelona (CDI), Barcelona, Spain

B. Díaz
Faculty of Medicine, University of Barcelona, Barcelona, Spain

Gynaecological Oncology Unit, Obstetrics and Gynaecology Department (ICGON), Hospital Clínic Barcelona, Barcelona, Spain

S. Vidal-Sicart (✉)
Nuclear Medicine, Hospital Clinic of Barcelona, Catalonia, Barcelona, Spain

Institut d'Investigacions Biomèdiques August Pi i Sunyer (IDIBAPS), Barcelona, Spain
e-mail: svidal@clinic.cat

1. Direct extension to adjacent structures (most common): The neoplasm originates from the surface epithelium. Since the endometrium is a monolayer epithelium, tumors can penetrate the myometrium relatively quickly, and eventually reach the serosa. The cervix, fallopian tubes, and finally the vagina and parametrium may be invaded. After complete penetration into and through the serosa, cells can spread along the pelvic lymphatics or into the peritoneal cavity or both (Fig. 4.1).
2. Transtubal passage of exfoliated cells: Tumor cells can be exfoliated from the primary tumor and transported to the peritoneal cavity by retrograde flow along the fallopian tubes. This route was suggested due to the detection of malignant cells in peritoneal lavages and the development of intra-abdominal metastases in some patients with early-stage endometrial cancer (Fig. 4.2).
3. Lymphatic dissemination: The lymphatic spread takes place along pelvic pathway. The three most important routes of dissemination in gynecologic neoplasms are the lateral, hypogastric, and presacral routes. However, in endometrial tumors the most important are the first two:
   (a) The lateral route drains lymph from the pelvic organs to the external iliac lymph node group.
   (b) The hypogastric route drains lymph along the visceral branches of the hypogastric vessels to the junctional lymph nodes (Fig. 4.3).

A. Collarino et al. (eds.), *Nuclear Medicine Manual on Gynaecological Cancers and Other Female Malignancies*, https://doi.org/10.1007/978-3-031-05497-6_4

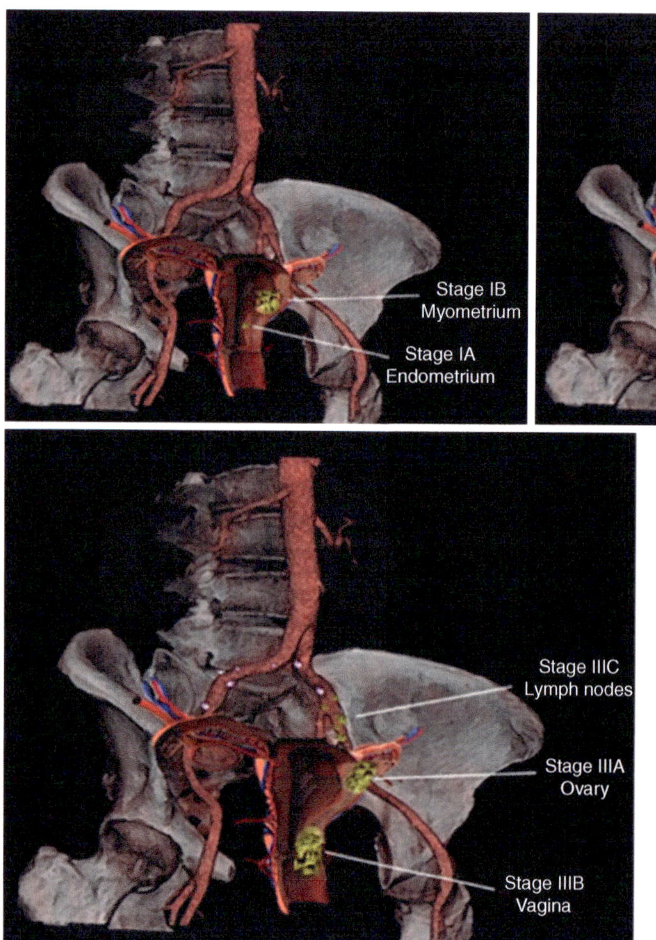

Fig. 4.1 Main routes of metastatic spread in endometrial cancer

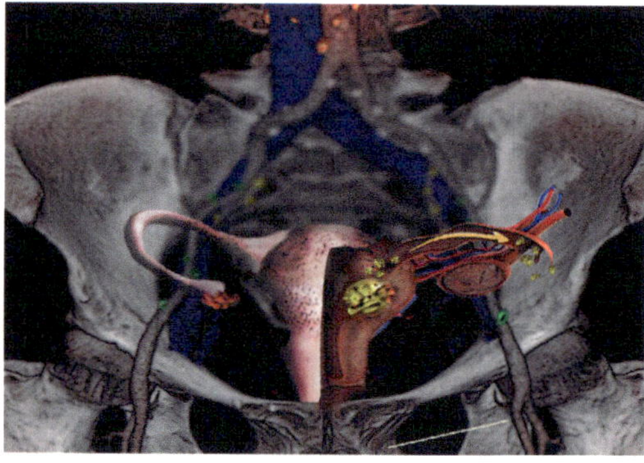

Fig. 4.2 Scheme of transtubal spreading of tumor cells

4. Hematogenous spread: Hematogenous metastases are not frequent. The lung and liver are the most commonly affected organs, as in other pelvic neoplasms.

4.1.2 Tumor Types

Histological types according to OMS 2014:

1. Endometrioid carcinoma of the endometrium (usual and variants)
2. Mucinous adenocarcinoma

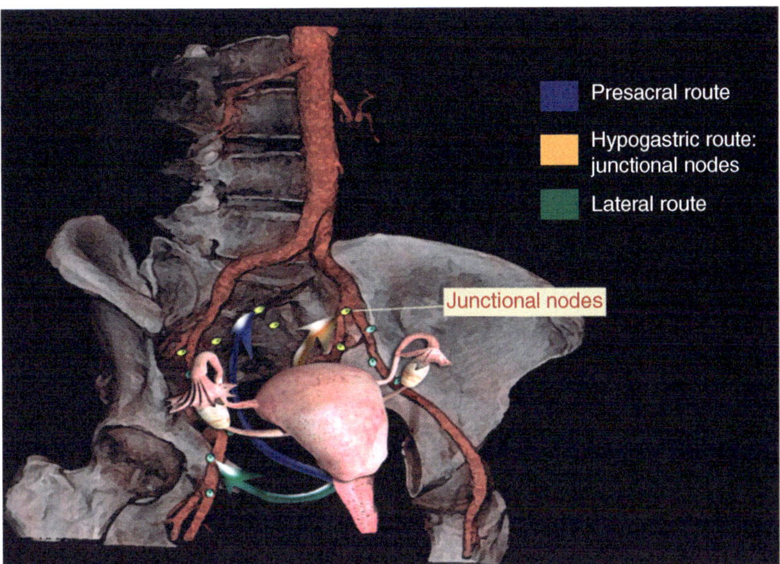

Fig. 4.3 Main lymphatic dissemination routes of endometrial cancer

3. Serous adenocarcinoma
4. Clear cell adenocarcinoma
5. Neuroendocrine tumors
6. Mixed adenocarcinoma
7. Undifferentiated and dedifferentiated carcinoma

Despite the fact that conventional pathological analysis remains an important tool for tumor classification, different groups have applied a diagnostic algorithm using three immunohistochemical markers (p53, MSH6, and PMS2) and a molecular test (exonuclease domain mutation analysis of POLE) to identify prognostic groups analogous to The Cancer Genomics Atlas (TCGA) molecular classification [1–3].

4.2 TNM-FIGO Classification

There are two systems used for staging endometrial cancer: the FIGO (International Federation of Gynaecology and Obstetrics) system, which is the most commonly used, and the AJCC (American Joint Committee on Cancer) TNM staging system (3).

Stage	TNM	FIGO stage	Stage description
I	T1 N0 M0	I	The cancer is found only in the uterus or womb. It may also be growing into the glands of the cervix, but not into the supporting connective tissue of the cervix (T1). It has not spread to nearby lymph nodes (N0) or to distant sites (M0).
IA	T1a N0 M0	IA	The cancer is found only in the endometrium or less than one-half of the myometrium (T1a). It has not spread to nearby lymph nodes (N0) or to distant sites (M0).
IB	T1b N0 M0	IB	The tumor has spread to one-half or more of the myometrium (T1b). It has not spread to nearby lymph nodes (N0) or to distant sites (M0).
II	T2 N0 M0	II	The tumor has spread from the uterus to the cervical stroma but not to other parts of the body. (T2). It has not spread to nearby lymph nodes (N0) or to distant sites (M0).
III	T3 N0 M0	III	The cancer has spread beyond the uterus, but it is still only in the pelvic area (T3). It has not spread to nearby lymph nodes (N0) or to distant sites (M0).

Stage	TNM	FIGO stage	Stage description
IIIA	T3a N0 M0	IIIA	The cancer has spread to the serosa of the uterus and/or the tissue of the fallopian tubes and ovaries but not to other parts of the body (T3a). It has not spread to nearby lymph nodes (N0) or to distant sites (M0).
IIIB	T3b N0 M0	IIIB	The cancer has spread to the vagina or to the paracervix (T3b). It has not spread to nearby lymph nodes (N0) or to distant sites (M0).
IIIC1	T1-T3 N1, N1mi or N1a M0	IIIC1	The cancer has spread to the regional pelvic lymph nodes (T1 to T3). It has also spread to pelvic lymph nodes (N1, N1mi, or N1a), but not to lymph nodes around the aorta or distant sites (M0).
IIIC2	T1-T3 N2, N2mi or N2a M0	IIIC2	The cancer has spread to the para-aortic lymph nodes (T1 to T3). It has also spread to lymph nodes around the aorta (para-aortic lymph nodes) (N2, N2mi, or N2a), but not to distant sites (M0).
IV	T4 Any N M0 or M1		The cancer has metastasized to the rectum, bladder, and/or distant organs.
IVA	T4 Any N M0		The cancer has spread to the mucosa of the rectum or bladder (T4). It may or may not have spread to nearby lymph nodes (Any N), but has not spread to distant sites (M0).
IVB	Any T Any N M1	IVB	The cancer has spread to lymph nodes in the groin area, and/or it has spread to distant organs, such as the bones or lungs (M1). The cancer can be any size (Any T) and it might or might not have spread to other lymph nodes (Any N).

4.3 Lymphatic Mapping (Sentinel Lymph Node)

4.3.1 Pathways of Lymphatic Spread (Expected Drainage)

The lymphatic drainage is complex: less orderly pattern than other tumors (less predictable!).

The pathway differs depending on the site of primary cancer. The pelvic pathway is the most common route (Fig. 4.4).

- Middle and lower aspects of the uterus: obturator lymph nodes (lateral route). MOST FREQUENTLY AFFECTED.
- Upper corpus and fundus: junctional lymph nodes (interiliac; hypogastric route)—common iliac lymph nodes—para-aortic.
- Fundus (less frequent): directly to para-aortic lymph nodes (para-aortic pathway, particularly left para-aortic lymph nodes at the level of the renal hilum) (Fig. 4.5).

4.3.2 Sentinel Lymph Node Biopsy

Indications

Pelvic lymph node dissection with or without para-aortic dissection is recommended, but sentinel lymph node (SLN) mapping can be considered due to the high sensitivity provided by ultrastaging. It has been widely studied in low-risk endometrial cancers defined by non-risk histologies (endometrioid), myometrial invasion <50%, and tumoral grade < G3.

The application in intermediate and high-risk EC is being investigated, although it is feasible. In this setting, the patients fulfill at least one of the following inclusion criteria: (1) Unfavorable histology (serous, clear cell, or grade 3 endometrioid adenocarcinoma); (2) myometrial invasion ≥50% suspected by imaging techniques (magnetic resonance imaging (MRI) or 3D ultrasound); (3) involvement of the cervical stroma confirmed by biopsy or suspected by imaging techniques.

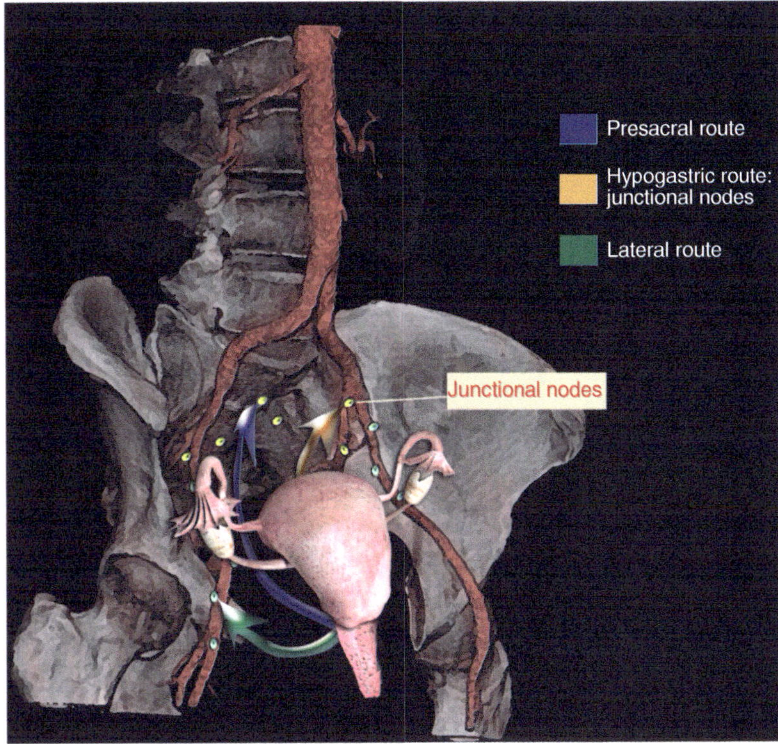

Fig. 4.4 Pelvic lymphatic routes of endometrial cancer spread

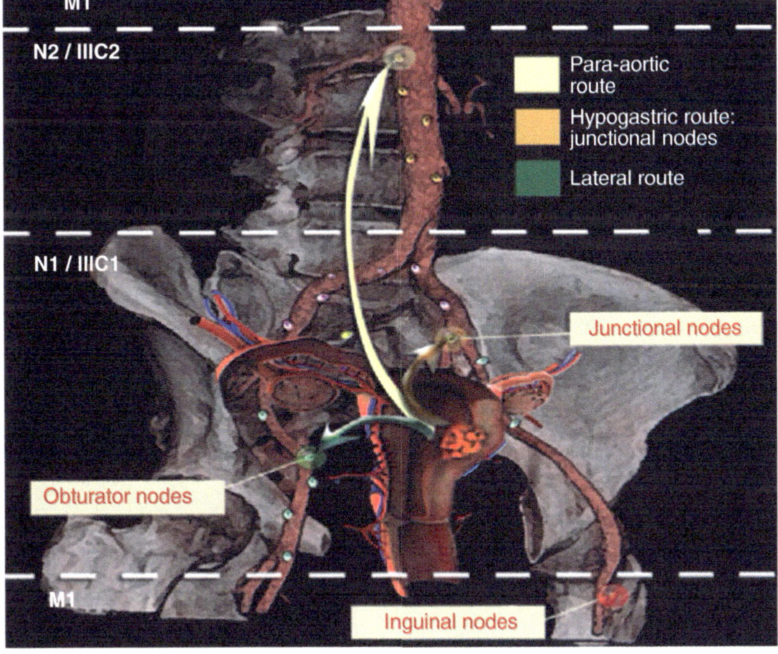

Fig. 4.5 Potential lymphatic routes of metastatic spread and their correlation with staging (N and M)

Patients and protocol must fulfil the next criteria:

- Stage I EC (distant metastases must be previously discarded).
- Nodal metastases must be excluded.
- In order to obtain a higher sensitivity, completion lymphadenectomy for unmapped sides is recommended (side-specific nodal dissection).
- Suspicious or enlarged nodes detected during surgery must be removed regardless of the lymphatic mapping.

Injection Sites

- Subserosal/fundal:
  - Detection rate: 73–89%.
  - Pros: high para-aortic SLN detection (30%).
  - Cons: no intraoperative image is available, risk of peritoneal spread of the tracer, needs to be performed during surgery.
- Myometrial:
  - Performed by hysteroscopy or by ultrasonography (TUMIR).
  - Detection rate 73–82%; bilaterality 37–40%.
  - Pros: the only injection site to provide a lymphatic map of para-aortic area.
  - Cons: lower total and bilateral detection rate; it requires an invasive procedure (hysteroscopic) or a skilled ultrasonographer (TUMIR).
- Cervical: It is the most common site of injection used (Fig. 4.6).
  - Detection rate: 87%.
  - Pros: easy to inject; available in all centers; high bilateral pelvic drainage (56–63%).
  - Cons: low rate of para-aortic drainage.

Combinations of cervical and myometrial/fundal injections have been evaluated, with an increase in the detection rate (60–86%) and bilaterality (60–94%).

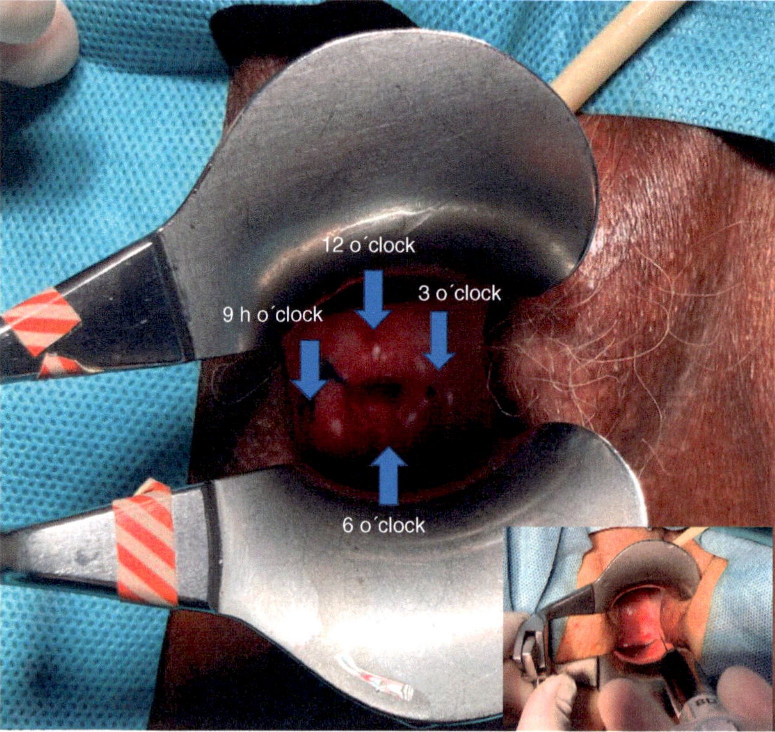

Fig. 4.6 Cervical injection of indocyanine green at 4 points around cervical external os

Tracers (Figs. 4.7 and 4.8)

- Blue dyes:
  - Pros: easy to inject, available in all centers.
  - Cons: lower detection rate than Indocyanine green (ICG), especially in women with high BMI; anaphylactic reactions can occur (1%); do not provide a preoperative image.
- Radiotracers.
  - Pros: provide a preoperative lymphatic mapping; higher sensitivity than blue dyes, no anaphylactic reactions; unexpected drainage can be detected.
  - Cons: need for a Nuclear Medicine Department/gamma-probe for intraoperative detection.
  - Radiotracer can be combined with other colorimetric tracers (blue dyes and/or ICG).
- ICG (indocyanine green).
  - Pros: highest sensitivity and NPV.
  - Cons: need for a near-infrared (NIR) camera; anaphylactic reactions (less than blue dyes), do not provide a preoperative lymphatic mapping.

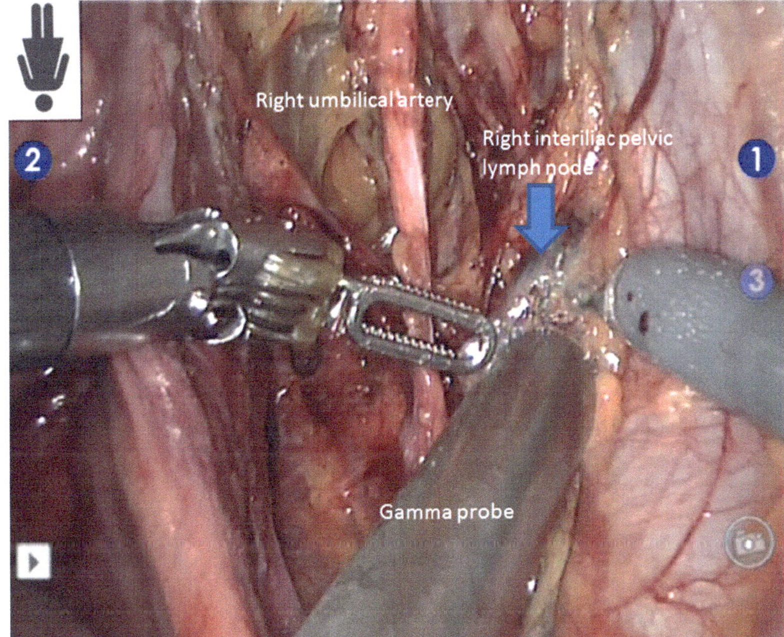

Fig. 4.7 Right interiliac pelvic lymph node detection detected by means of a gamma-probe (radiotracer activity) and after blue dye injection

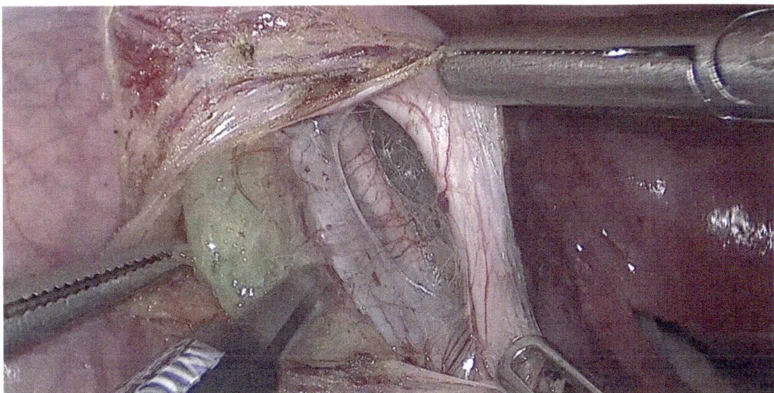

Fig. 4.8 Intraoperative SLN (hybrid tracer ICG-[^{99m}Tc]Tc-albumin nanocolloid) detection with a near-infrared camera

Blue dyes are not recommended to be used alone for EC SLN due to their lower intraoperative detection rate. Hybrid tracers combine radiotracers and ICG in a single tracer with higher sensitivity than radiotracers alone [1, 4–7].

4.4 Utility of SPECT/CT

The information provided by SPECT/CT has demonstrated to increase in the number of SLNs identified and, more relevantly, the number of lymphatic chains with drainage. Preoperative imaging provides important information about drainage in expected and unexpected areas, which is essential to guide the surgeon during intraoperative SLN detection. Therefore, it is an essential tool in sentinel node detection of malignancies with pelvic drainage such as endometrial cancer, especially when non-cervical injection is performed. The use of Maximum Intensity Projection (MIP) to display fused SPECT/CT images may help surgeons anatomically recognize and localize radioactive targets. The anatomical localization of lesions with radiotracer uptake does transform SPECT/CT in interventional imaging. Surgeons can use the provided anatomical landmarks (blood vessels, muscles, and other structures) to retrieve these targets during operation (Figs. 4.9, 4.10 and 4.11).

The benefits of SPECT/CT vs. planar lymphoscintigraphy can be summarized in:

- Increases the detection rate against planar lymphoscintigraphy or blue dyes:
  - 77–84% vs. 67–68% (planar lymphoscintigraphy)
  - 90% vs. 80% (blue dye).
- Detection rate similar to gamma-probe (90% vs. 88%) and ICG.
- Increases the number of regions with drainage/bilaterality: 43–53% vs. 32–39%.
- Increases the detection of atypical drainage: 37% vs. 16%.

The main acquisition characteristics for SPECT/CT are summarized in the following table. It must be taken into consideration, that the values are orientative and they should be adjusted depending on every device and physician's preferences.

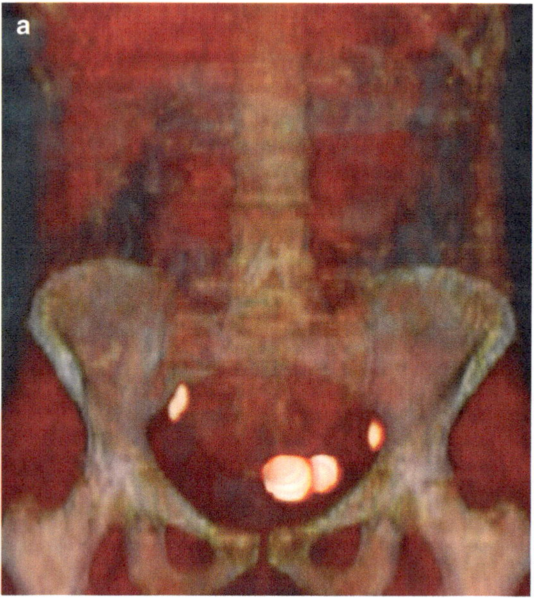

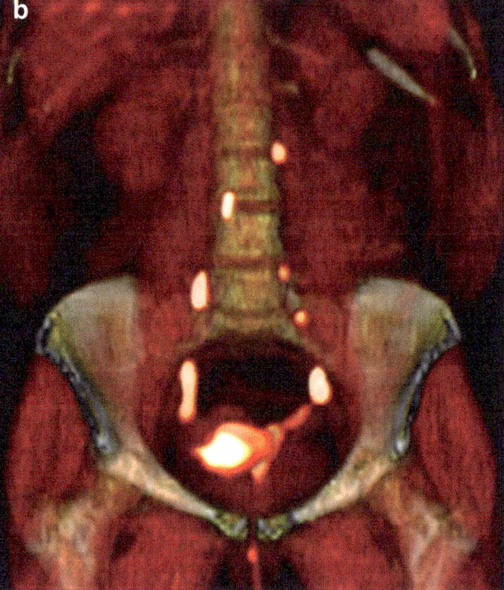

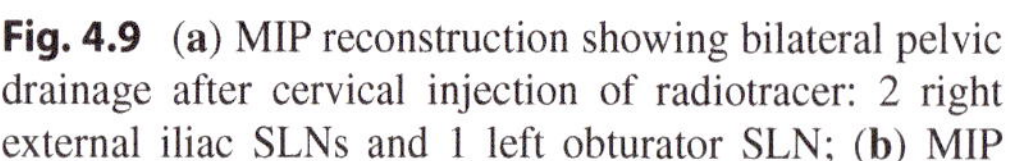

Fig. 4.9 (**a**) MIP reconstruction showing bilateral pelvic drainage after cervical injection of radiotracer: 2 right external iliac SLNs and 1 left obturator SLN; (**b**) MIP reconstruction showing bilateral pelvic and para-aortic drainage after myometrial injection of radiotracer

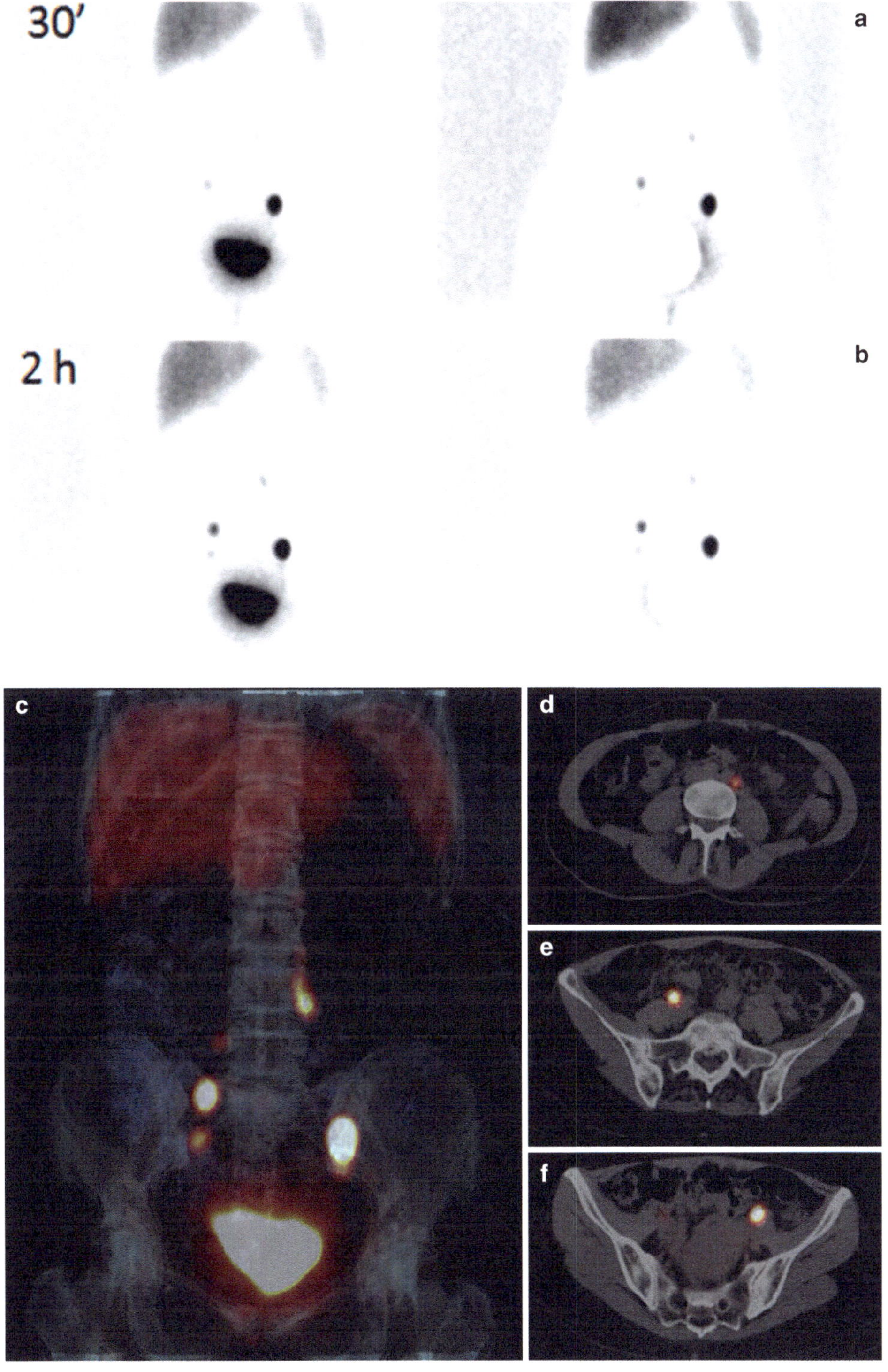

Fig. 4.10 Early planar images showing bilateral drainage at 30 min (**a**), with increased uptake on the delayed images (**b**) after cervical injection of radiotracer. MIP image from SPECT/CT (**c**) shows the same drainage and axial fused SPECT/CT slices (**d**–**f**) show a left common iliac, as the most cranial SLN (**d**), a right common iliac (**e**), and a right interiliac SLNs

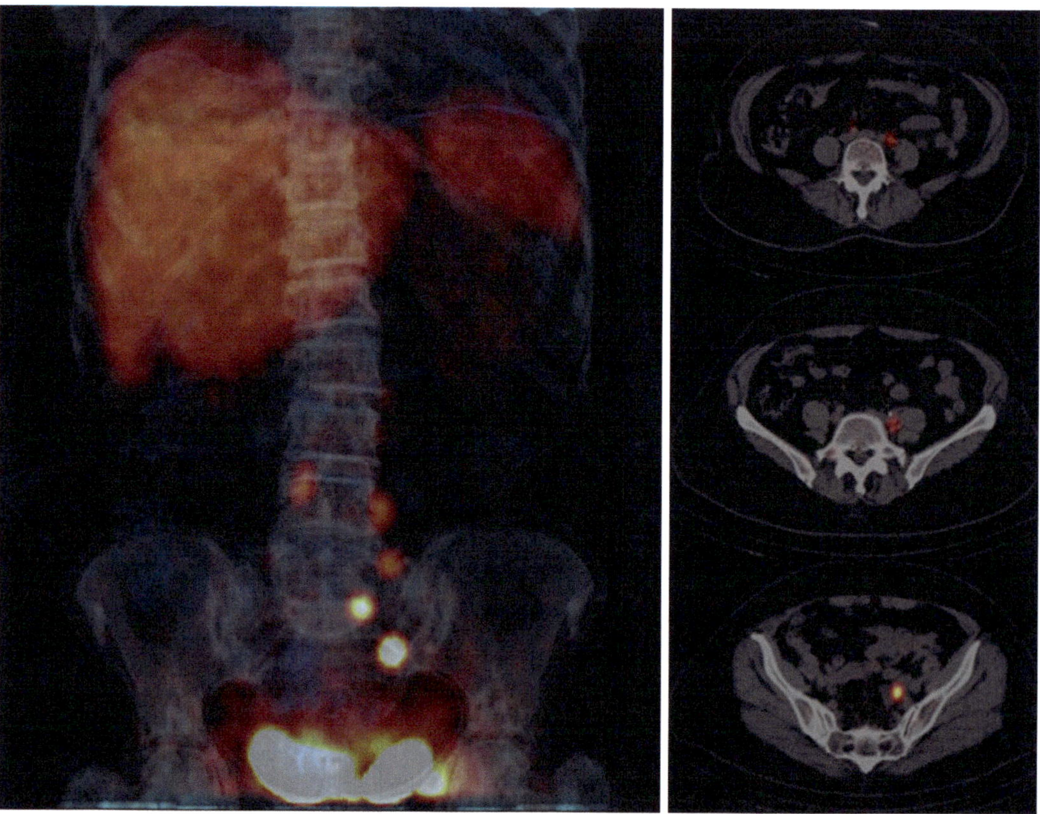

Fig. 4.11 MIP image from SPECT/CT (C) showing bilateral drainage (right common iliac node and left common iliac, presacral, and hypogastric nodes)

Methodology

Acquisition parameters	
Projections	120 (60 per head)
Orbit	360° non circular
Acquisition time	30 s/step
Matrix (SPECT)	128 × 128 matrix
Pixel size	Pixel size 3.30 × 3.30 mm^2
Energy photopeak	130 keV–151 keV
Energy window for scatter correction	110 keV–130 keV
CT for attenuation correction and fusion – Matrix – Energy	– 512 × 512 – 130 KV and 2.5 mAs
Reconstruction	OSEM: 5 subsets, 20 iterations Gaussian filter (FWHM 6 mm)

Interpretation

Images should be accurately revised by an experienced nuclear medicine physician in radioguided surgery. The image threshold must be modified to avoid background activity coming from the injection site in order to isolate each hot spot with its different activity. Findings must be reported as the number of sentinel lymph nodes detected and the relation with vessels (number of echelon nodes). It is strongly recommended to discuss the findings with the surgical team previous to surgery [8–12] (Fig. 4.12).

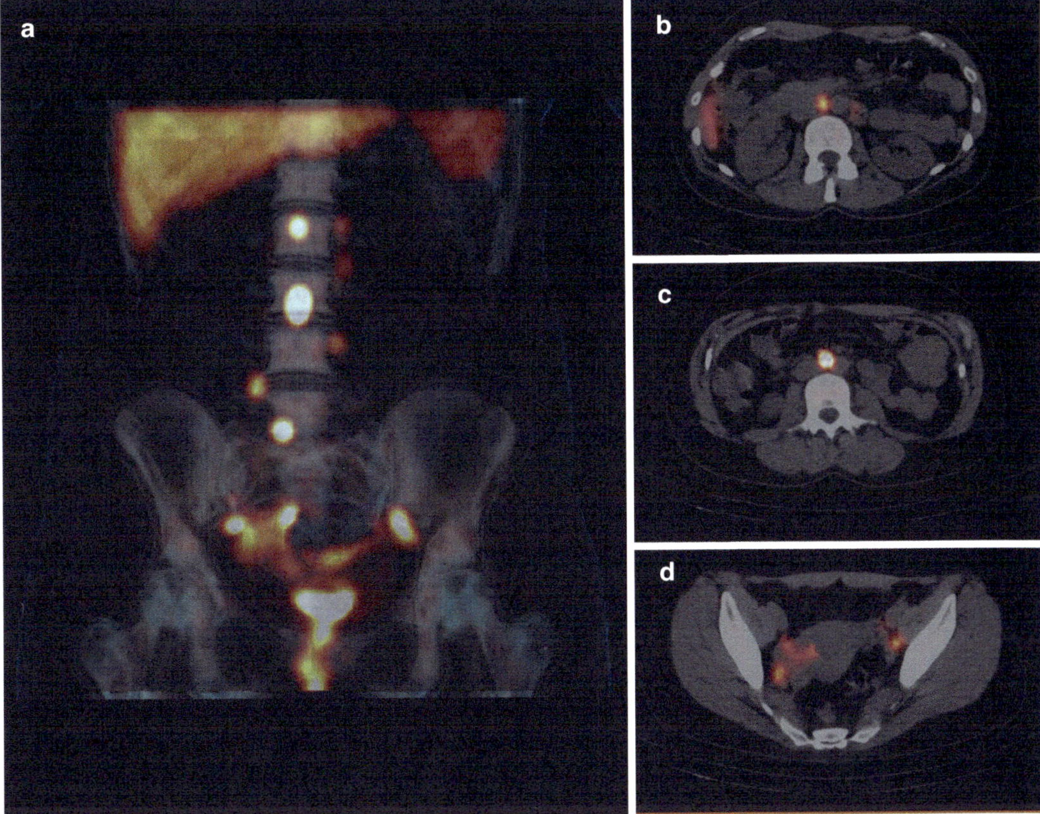

Fig. 4.12 Bilateral pelvic plus para-aortic drainage after myometrial injection of hybrid tracer ([99mTc] Tc-albumin colloid) in a 62-year-old woman affected with serous endometrial carcinoma. (**a**) MIP image showing bilateral pelvic drainage, para-aortic and interaortocaval SLNs. (**b–d**) Axial fused images from SPECT/CT: interaortocaval SLNs (**b–c**) and bilateral external SLNs (**d**). Right iliac external SLN (arrow) nearby injection site is clearly differentiated on CT

4.5 Utility of MRI and PET/CT

4.5.1 Role of Morphologic Imaging Techniques in Staging

The technique of choice for staging is MR imaging, since it assists in preoperative assessment and surgical planning by helping predict the depth of myometrial invasion, cervical involvement, distant spread, and lymph node involvement (Fig. 4.13).

Lymph node metastasis is the most common form of extrauterine disease spread.

Several studies have found that lymph node involvement is a strong predictor of recurrence and survival, and its presence warrants upstaging to stage IIIC disease.

The probability of metastatic lymph node involvement is greater in patients with:

- High-grade lesions at cytologic analysis.
- Lympho-vascular space involvement.
- Myometrial invasion to a depth of over 50%.
- Cervical infiltration.

According to the latest guidelines of the European Society of Urogenital Radiology (ESUR) regarding the staging of endometrial neoplasms with MR imaging, imaging signs of lymph node involvement include a short-axis

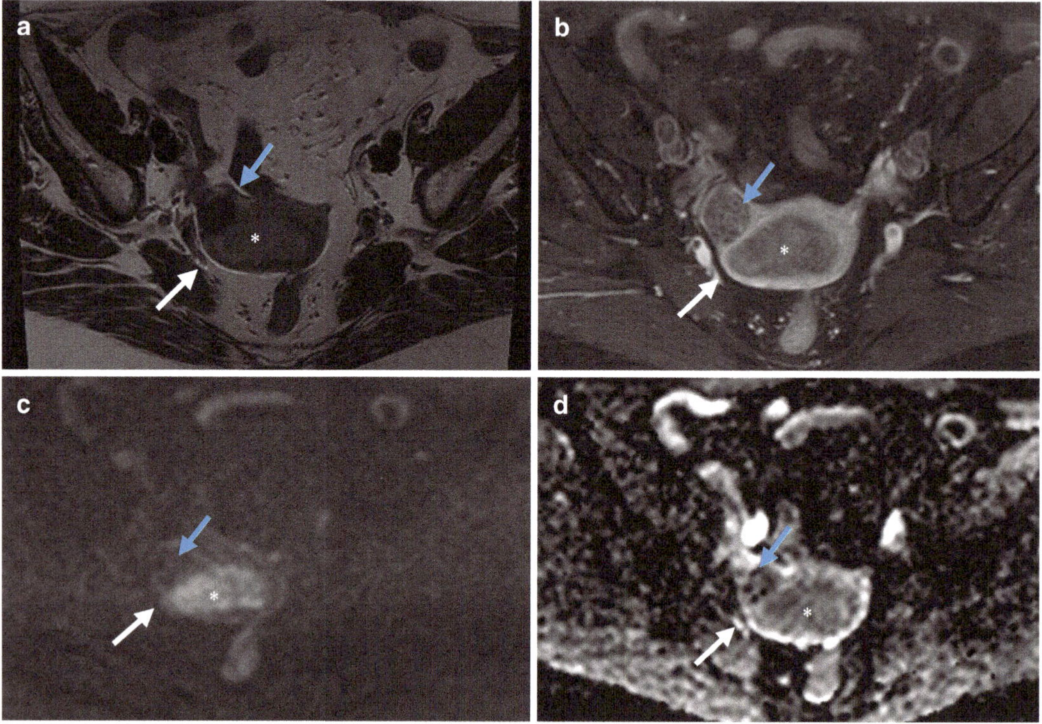

Fig. 4.13 A 73-year-old female with postmenopausal bleeding. MRI in axial plane T2 (**a**), T1 Fatsat with contrast (**b**), DWI (b 800) (**c**), and ADC (**d**) sequences showing 38 × 22 mm endometrial mass that occupies almost the entire cavity (*) with signs of infiltration at the right posterolateral and cornual level, where the distance from the serosa is approx. 2–3 mm, which suggests focal myometrial infiltration greater than 50% (White arrow). Right cornual subserous myoma 4 cm (blue arrow). No signs of lymph node or intra-abdominal spread

diameter of at least 8 mm for nodes in the pelvis and more than 10 mm for nodes in the retroperitoneum, especially in the presence of another nodal characteristic suggestive of involvement, such as a round appearance or necrosis.

However, diagnosing lymph node involvement with MR imaging has a low sensitivity of 50% in the detection of affected adenopathies, with a specificity of 95%.

4.5.2 Role of Functional Imaging Techniques in Staging ([^{18}F]FDG-PET/CT)

Normal uptake of [^{18}F]FDG in the endometrium varies depending on the menstrual phase (in premenopausal women), with an increasing uptake during menstrual but also ovulatory phases. Dating the last menstrual period (LMP) is necessary to correctly interpret the findings. An increased uptake outside this range must be studied by transvaginal ultrasonography. Benign conditions can show high [^{18}F]FDG uptake: uterine myomas, endometriosis, and salpingitis.

[^{18}F]FDG uptake differs from each histology, being the endometrial carcinoma the most hypermetabolic histology and leiomyosarcoma the least. So, it is not recommended to lesion characterization. Other tracers such as fluoroestradiol ([^{18}F]FES), as an estrogen receptor tracer, are highly expressed in high-risk endometrial carcinoma. However, endometrial can-

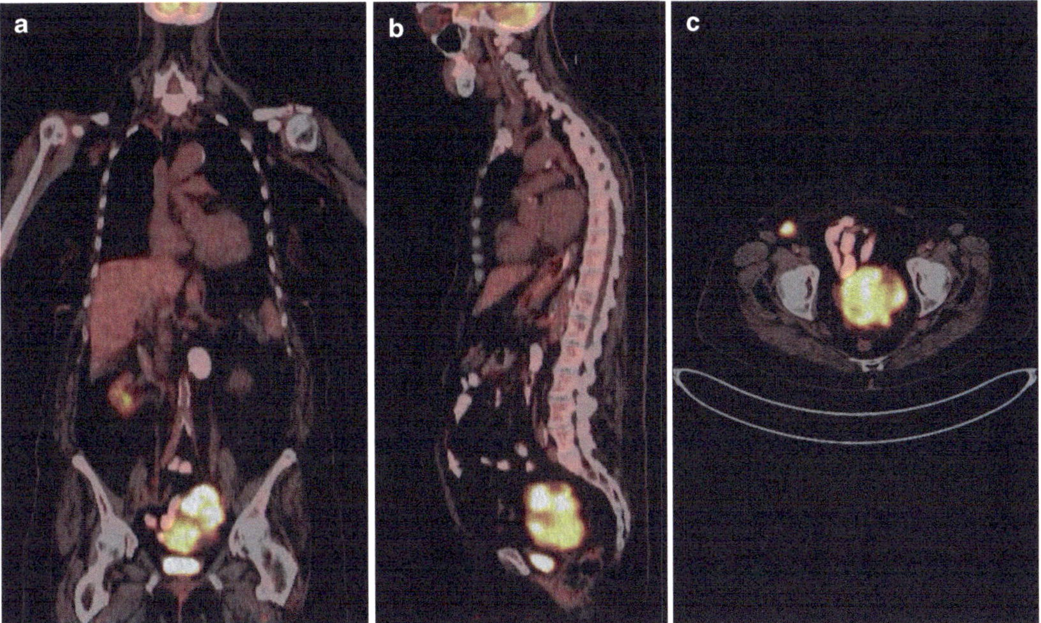

Fig. 4.14 FDG-PET/CT study in a 84-year-old woman with several comorbidities in whom surgical nodal staging was discarded. Coronal (**a**), sagittal (**b**), and axial (**c**) views showing endometrial primary cancer and right inguinal nodes

cer staging can be assessed by [^{18}F]FDG-PET/CT to identify lymph node and distant metastasis, up to 12% of cases in high-risk endometrial carcinoma (Fig. 4.14). Sensitivity for nodal staging is low when the microscopical disease is considered, but negative predictive value achieves 94%.

Indications

- Endometrial cancer in advanced stages for staging purposes.
- High-risk endometrial cancer in early stage when surgical nodal staging is not achieved.
- Radiation treatment planning (optional).
- Detection of recurrence (it is not recommended as an imaging tool during surveillance).
- Response assessment (optional).

Methodology

Low-dose PET/CT offers high performance for staging purposes, but contrast-enhanced CT is preferred for the detection of peritoneal carcinomatosis. Coronal and sagittal abdominal reconstructions are crucial for staging purposes.

Oral contrast is useful to discriminate bowel physiological uptake from peritoneal implants.

If performed for radiation treatment planning purposes, consider positioning the patient on a flat radiation therapy pallet, with no bed overlapping and no use of contrast agents [13–17] (Figs. 4.15 and 4.16).

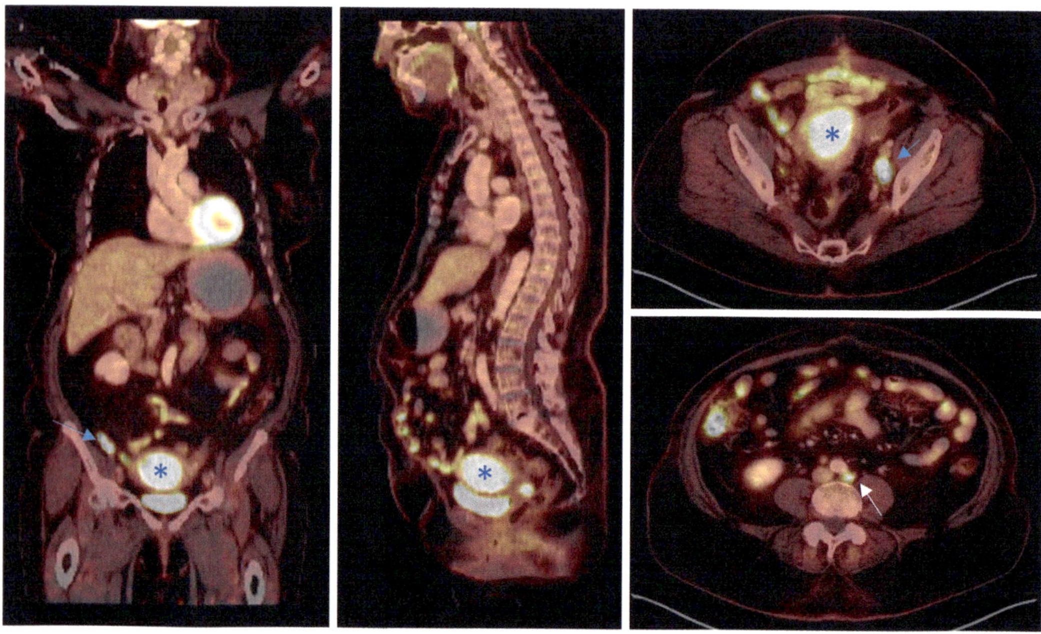

Fig. 4.15 A 67-year-old woman with grade 3 endometrioid endometrial cancer. [^{18}F]FDG-PET/CT shows primary tumor (blue asterisk) with nodal spreading through pelvic chains, bilateral external (blue arrows), and internal iliac nodes as well as para-aortic nodal involvement (white arrow)

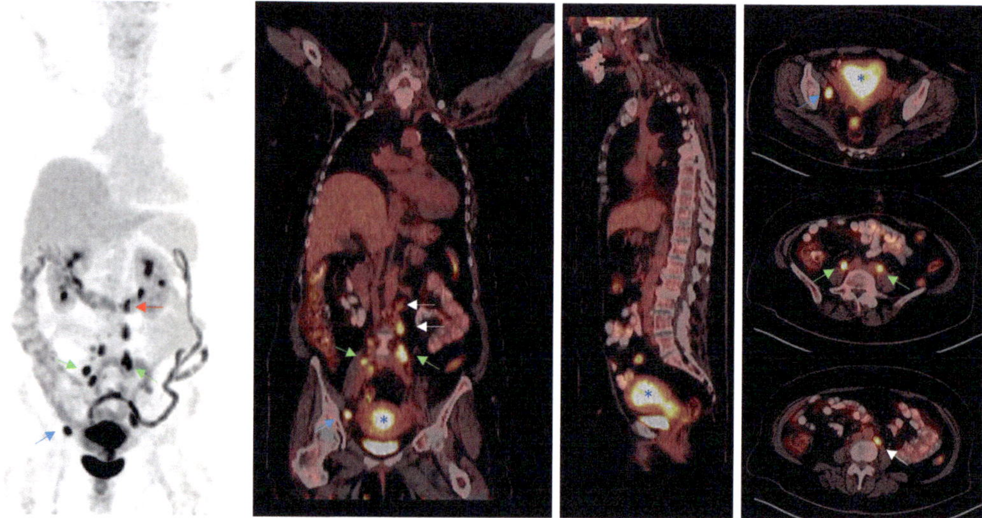

Fig. 4.16 A 67-year-old woman with endometrioid endometrial cancer involving the cervix (blue asterisk) with nodal spreading through pelvic chains, bilateral external (blue arrows), and internal iliac nodes as well as para-aortic nodal involvement (white arrow). Bilateral pelvic and para-aortic nodal involvement is detected on [^{18}F]FDG-PET/CT in the right external iliac region (blue arrows), both common iliac chains (green arrows) and para-aortic nodes (white and red arrows)

4.6 ROLL and/or RSL for Non-palpable Lesions Recurrence

Radioguided surgery technique has been successfully used in several clinical indications based on the accumulation of an injected radiotracer in a target lesion that is designed to be retained at the injection site (ROLL; Radioguided Occult Lesion Localization; RSL: Radioguided Seed Localization).

In ROLL approach, part of the tracer used for sentinel lymph node biopsy is retained inside the lesion (if intratumorally injected) and it can be used to demarcate the primary lesion or its margins. The most used approach is the use of [99mTc]Tc-macroaggregate albumin (MAA), with a high particle size, that avoid its lymphatic spread and can improve the local tracer retention.

Indications

This approach has served as alternative to other options, like hook-wire, needles…., for marking the non-palpable or occult lesions with a high reliability.

Advantages

- The radiotracer can be injected into the lesion the day before or some hours prior to surgery without losing the capacity for lesion localization. This technique allows location of the lesion guided by a gamma detector probe (used in sentinel node).
- Reduction of dose of exposure to ionizing radiations among surgical personnel since ROLL generates exposure of 1/5000 of the dose permitted to hands and is lower than the dosimetry accepted for the public.
- Flexibility of surgical schedule.
- Shorter surgical time (one activity focus without radioactive background).

Disadvantages

- Tracer spreading (larger tissue resections)
- Non-accessible lesions to be injected (avoids technique)
- Non-nodular lesions (tracer diffusion)

Methodological Aspects for Injection (CT-Guided) and Resection (Probes, Other Devices…)

- Check the lesion in previous diagnostic images (CT, MRI, ultrasound, PET/CT).
- -Decide which imaging technique will be used for radiotracer injection (usually ultrasound or CT) and confirm the correct lesion localization.
- -Calculating the shortest distance between the skin and nodule while taking into account the tissues that will be passed through.
- A slow injection of 0.1–0.2 mL of [99mTc]Tc-MAA (37–74 MBq, depending on the day of injection) is given (Fig. 4.17).
- 0.2 mL of radiopaque contrast medium or 0.1–0.3 mL of air (for needle lavage) can be given.
- Verification of the administration may be carried out in two ways:
  - An image verifies that the contrast medium (if used) is in place.
  - The most used approach is performing a scintigraphic image (ideally with SPECT/CT) to rule out the potential tracer spillage.
- A skin mark could be helpful in some lesions (especially superficial).
- During surgery (open or laparoscopic) the gamma-probe must be strategically placed and an accurate scanning of the zone should

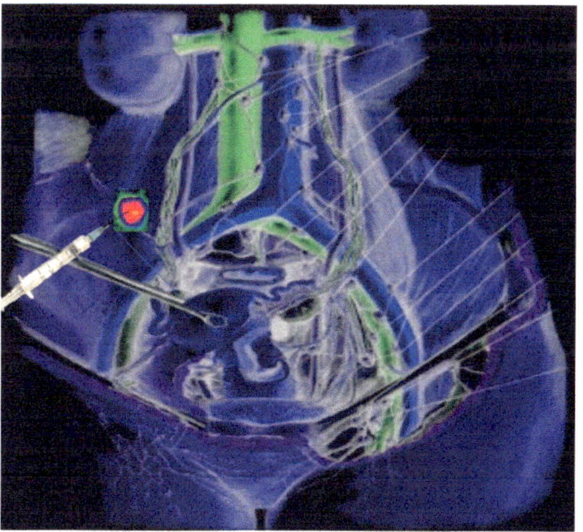

Fig. 4.17 Scheme about ROLL technique in a right iliac lesion. Locally injection of radiotracer (guided by CT or ultrasound) in the right pelvic area where a solitary metastasis from endometrial cancer has grown

be performed to identify the focus of greatest radioactivity.

- After removal of lesion, absence of residual activity in the surgical field should be confirmed [18–22].

Radioguided Seed Localization

This procedure uses a sealed titanium capsule (4 × 0.8 mm) that fits within a 18-G needle containing a nontherapeutic low dose of 125I (usually 7 MBq). RSL has mostly been applied in breast cancer patients for tumor resection (like ROLL) and, especially in those receiving neoadjuvant treatment.

Advantages

- Sealed radioactive source (no spillage).
- Flexibility in surgery timing (from several to same-day prior to surgery).
- Low radiation.
- Improved definition of the incision site.
- High reliability of intraoperative target detection.

Disadvantages

- Regulatory issues.
- Potential loss of the seed.
- Not always possible to be introduced into the lesion.

Methodological aspects for injection (CT-guided) and resection (probes, other devices…)

- Check the lesion in previous diagnostic images (CT, MRI, ultrasound, PET/CT).
- Decide which imaging technique will be a need for injection (ultrasound or CT) and confirm the correct lesion localization.
- Calculating the shortest distance between the skin and nodule while taking into account the tissues that will be passed through.
- A 18-gauge needle, long enough for the injection is used. The tip of the needle is covered by bone wax (to avoid seed's fall).
- Continuous monitoring with ultrasound probe (or CT control) is performed (Fig. 4.18).

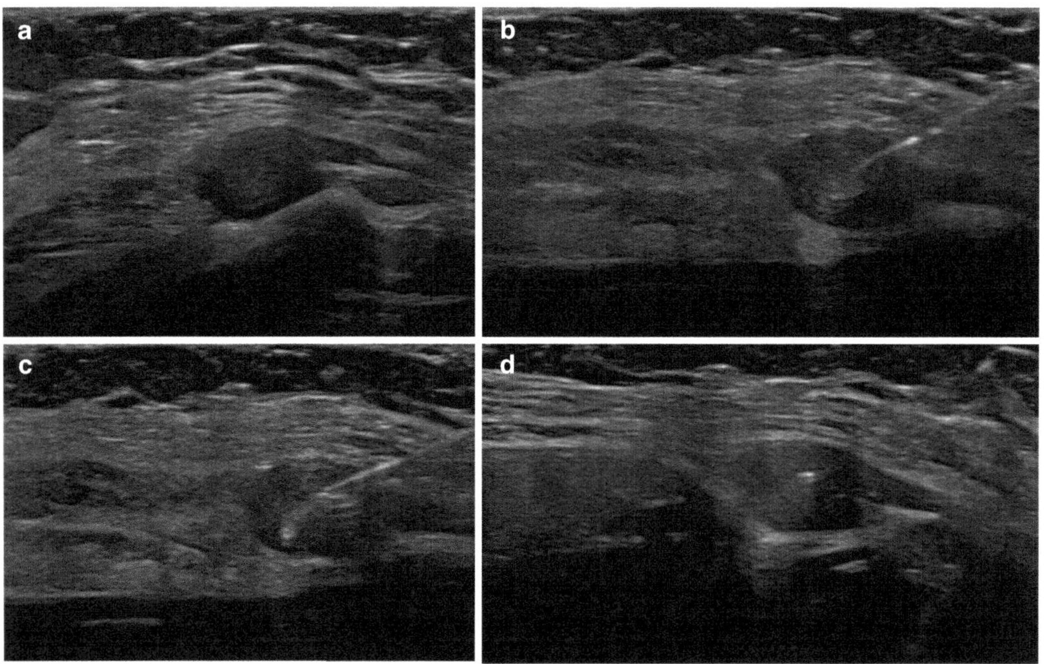

Fig. 4.18 RSL approach. A superficial inguinal node is well depicted with ultrasound image (**a**). A 18-G needle is inserted into the center of the lesion (**b**). A ^{125}I seed is deployed within the nodule (**c**). After withdrawal of the needle, the seed is clearly visualized into the lesion (**d**)

- When needle's tip position is adequate the guide of the needle is pushed in order to release the seed.
- Verification of the administration may be carried out by on-site ultrasound or radiologic image. Moreover, a scintigraphic image with a gamma camera is usually done (set up in 27 KeV energy photopeak). With these images the adequate seed position into the lesion is checked (especially in SPECT/CT fused images).
- A skin mark could be helpful in some lesions (especially superficial).
- During surgery (open or laparoscopic) the gamma-probe (with isotope selection set at ^{125}I energy) should perform a detailed scanning to identify the focus of radioactivity.
- Once localized, the surgeon dissects the tissues and nuclear medicine staff verifies with the probe that the radioactive focus is properly addressed.
- Absence of residual activity in the surgical field should be confirmed [23–27]

References

1. Concin N, Matias-Guiu X, Vergote I, Cibula D, Mirza MR, Marnitz S, Ledermann J, Bosse T, Chargari C, Fagotti A, Fotopoulou C, Gonzalez Martin A, Lax S, Lorusso D, Marth C, Morice P, Nout RA, O'Donnell D, Querleu D, Raspollini MR, Sehouli J, Sturdza A, Taylor A, Westermann A, Wimberger P, Colombo N, Planchamp F, Creutzberg CL. ESGO/ESTRO/ESP guidelines for the management of patients with endometrial carcinoma. Int J Gynecol Cancer. 2021;31:12–39. https://doi.org/10.1136/ijgc-2020-002230.
2. Murali R, Soslow RA, Weigelt B. Classification of endometrial carcinoma: more than two types. Lancet Oncol. 2014;15:e268–78. https://doi.org/10.1016/S1470-2045(13)70591-6.
3. WHO Classification of Tumours. Female genital organ tumours, international agency for research on cancer IARC. 5th edn. Lyon, 2020.
4. Abu-Rustum, NR; Yashar, CM; Bradley, K; Campos, SM; Chon, HS; Chu C et al. NCCN Guidelines. Uterine Neoplasms Version 1.2021.
5. Giammarile F, Bozkurt MF, Cibula D, Pahisa J, Oyen WJ, Paredes P, Olmos RV, Sicart SV. The EANM clinical and technical guidelines for lymphoscintigraphy and sentinel node localization in gynaecological cancers. Eur J Nucl Med Mol Imaging. 2014;41:1463–77. https://doi.org/10.1007/s00259-014-2732-8.
6. Martinelli F, Ditto A, Bogani G, Leone Roberti Maggiore U, Signorelli M, Chiappa V, Raspagliesi F. Sentinel lymph node mapping in endometrial cancer: performance of hysteroscopic injection of tracers. Int J Gynecol Cancer. 2020;30:332–8. https://doi.org/10.1136/ijgc-2019-000930.
7. Skanjeti A, Dhomps A, Paschetta C, Tordo J, Giammarile F. Sentinel node mapping in gynecologic cancers: a comprehensive review. Semin Nucl Med. 2019;49:521–33. https://doi.org/10.1053/j.semnuclmed.2019.06.012.
8. Belhocine TZ, Prefontaine M, Lanvin D, Bertrand M, Rachinsky I, Ettler H, Zabel P, Stitt LW, Sugimoto A, Urbain JL. Added-value of SPECT/CT to lymphatic mapping and sentinel lymphadenectomy in gynaecological cancers. Am J Nucl Med Mol Imaging. 2013;3:182–93.
9. Buda A, Elisei F, Arosio M, Dolci C, Signorelli M, Perego P, Giuliani D, Recalcati D, Cattoretti G, Milani R, Messa C. Integration of hybrid single-photon emission computed tomography/computed tomography in the preoperative assessment of sentinel node in patients with cervical and endometrial cancer: our experience and literature review. Int J Gynecol Cancer. 2012;22:830–5. https://doi.org/10.1097/IGC.0b013e318253496f.
10. Elisei F, Crivellaro C, Giuliani D, Dolci C, De Ponti E, Montanelli L, La Manna M, Guerra L, Arosio M, Landoni C, Buda A. Sentinel-node mapping in endometrial cancer patients: comparing SPECT/CT, gamma-probe and dye. Ann Nucl Med. 2017;31:93–9. https://doi.org/10.1007/s12149-016-1137-0.
11. Navarro AS, Angeles MA, Migliorelli F, Illac C, Martínez-Gómez C, Leray H, Betrian S, Chantalat E, Tanguy Le Gac Y, Motton S, Querleu D, Ferron G, Gabiache E, Martinez A. Comparison of SPECT-CT with intraoperative mapping in cervical and uterine malignancies. Int J Gynecol Cancer. 2021;31(679–685) https://doi.org/10.1136/ijgc-2020-002198.
12. Togami S, Kawamura T, Yanazume S, Kamio M, Kobayashi H. Comparison of lymphoscintigraphy and single photon emission computed tomography with computed tomography (SPECT/CT) for sentinel lymph node detection in endometrial cancer. Int J Gynecol Cancer. 2020;30:626–30. https://doi.org/10.1136/ijgc-2019-001154.
13. Bollineni VR, Ytre-Hauge S, Bollineni-Balabay O, Salvesen HB, Haldorsen IS. High diagnostic value of 18F-FDG PET/CT in endometrial cancer: systematic review and meta-analysis of the literature. J Nucl Med. 2016 Jun;57:879–85. https://doi.org/10.2967/jnumed.115.170597.
14. Lerman H, Metser U, Grisaru D, Fishman A, Lievshitz G, Even-Sapir E. Normal and abnormal 18F-FDG endometrial and ovarian uptake in pre- and postmenopausal patients: assessment by PET/CT. J Nucl Med. 2004;45:266–71.
15. Park JY, Kim EN, Kim DY, Suh DS, Kim JH, Kim YM, Kim YT, Nam JH. Comparison of the validity of magnetic resonance imaging and positron emis-

sion tomography/computed tomography in the preoperative evaluation of patients with uterine corpus cancer. Gynecol Oncol. 2008;108:486–92. https://doi.org/10.1016/j.ygyno.2007.11.044.
16. Taşkin S, Varli B, Ersöz CC, Altin D, Soydal Ç, Ortaç F. Complementary role of 18F-FDG PET/CT for sentinel lymph node algorithm in endometrial cancer with high-risk factors for lymphatic metastasis. Nucl Med Commun. 2020;41:389–94. https://doi.org/10.1097/MNM.0000000000001157.
17. Tsuyoshi H, Tsujikawa T, Yamada S, Okazawa H, Yoshida Y. Diagnostic value of 18F-FDG PET/MRI for staging in patients with endometrial cancer. Cancer Imaging. 2020;20(1):75. https://doi.org/10.1186/s40644-020-00357-4.
18. Bowles H, Sánchez N, Tapias A, Paredes P, Campos F, Bluemel C, Valdés Olmos RA, Vidal-Sicart S. Radioguided surgery and the GOSTT concept: from pre- operative image and intraoperative navigation to image-assisted excision. Rev Esp Med Nucl Imagen Mol. 2017;36:175–84. https://doi.org/10.1016/j.remn.2016.09.004.
19. Landman J, Kulawansa S, McCarthy M, Troedson R, Phillips M, Tinning J, Taylor D. Radioguided localisation of impalpable breast lesions using 99m-technetium macroaggregated albumin: lessons learnt during introduction of a new technique to guide preoperative localisation. J Med Radiat Sci. 2015;62:6–14. https://doi.org/10.1002/jmrs.36.
20. Manca G, Garau LM, Romanini A, Rubello D, Nuzzo A, Barbarello L, Fantechi L, Colletti PM, Boggi U, Volterrani D. Detection of uterine Leiomyosarcoma peritoneal lesions by SPECT/CT and ROLL technique. Clin Nucl Med. 2019;44:826–8. https://doi.org/10.1097/RLU.0000000000002725.
21. Manca G, Mazzarri S, Rubello D, Tardelli E, Delgado-Bolton RC, Giammarile F, Roncella M, Volterrani D, CollettiPM. Radioguided occult lesion localization: technical procedures and clinical applications. Clin Nucl Med. 2017;42:e498–503. https://doi.org/10.1097/RLU.0000000000001858.
22. Vidal-Sicart S, Fuertes Cabero S, Danús Lainez M, Valdés Olmos R, Paredes Barranco P, Rayo Madrid JI, Rioja Martín ME, Díaz Expósito R, Goñi GE. Update on radioguided surgery: from international consensus on sentinel node in head and neck cancer to the advances on gynaecological tumors and localization of non-palpable lesions. Rev Esp Med Nucl Imagen Mol. 2019;38:173–82. https://doi.org/10.1016/j.remn.2020.11.003.
23. Garner HW, Bestic JM, Peterson JJ, Attia S, Wessell DE. Preoperative radioactive seed localization of nonpalpable soft tissue masses: an established localization technique with a new application. Skelet Radiol. 2017;46:209–16. https://doi.org/10.1007/s00256-016-2529-x.
24. Hassing CMS, Tvedskov TF, Kroman N, Klausen TL, Drejøe JB, Tvedskov JF, Lambine TL, Kledal H, Lelkaitis G, Langhans L. Radioactive seed localisation of non-palpable lymph nodes - a feasibility study. Eur J Surg Oncol. 2018;44:725–30. https://doi.org/10.1016/j.ejso.2018.02.211.
25. Jakub J, Gray R. Starting a radioactive seed localization program. Ann Surg Oncol. 2015;22:3197–202. https://doi.org/10.1245/s10434-015-4719-5.
26. Ng AH, Alqahtani MS, Jambi LK, Bugby SL, Lees JE, Perkins AC. Assessing a small field of view hybrid gamma camera for perioperative iodine-125 seed localisation. Br J Radiol. 2019;92(1098):20190020. https://doi.org/10.1259/bjr.20190020.
27. Valdés Olmos RA, Vidal-Sicart S, Manca G, Mariani G, León-Ramírez LF, Rubello D, Giammarile F. Advances in radioguided surgery in oncology. Q J Nucl Med Mol Imaging. 2017;61:247–70. https://doi.org/10.23736/S1824-4785.17.02995-8.

5 Ovarian Cancer

Berta Díaz, Blanca Paño, Pilar Paredes, and Sergi Vidal-Sicart

5.1 General Aspects

5.1.1 Anatomy

Lymphatic drainage of the ovary is much more complex than the one observed in the cervix, vulva, or breast. The double ovarian vascularization that accompanies lymphatic drainage explains this higher complexity. Vascularization of the ovary is formed by: (1) ovarian arteries, coming from the supramesenteric aorta, and ovarian veins that drain into the left renal cava and vein (both reach the ovary through the pelvic infundibular ligament) and (2) complimentary circulation of the ovary from the uterine vessels (branches of the internal iliac artery and vein) that reach the ovary through the utero-ovarian ligament. Therefore, the lymphatic drainage territory of the ovary includes the entire retroperitoneum from the inguinal ligament (caudal) to the left renal vein (cranial). It is unpredictable to know which will be the lymph node dissemination pathway of each lesion in a particular case, which makes it necessary to obtain a lymphatic map prior to the intraoperative detection of sentinel lymph node (SLN) (Fig. 5.1).

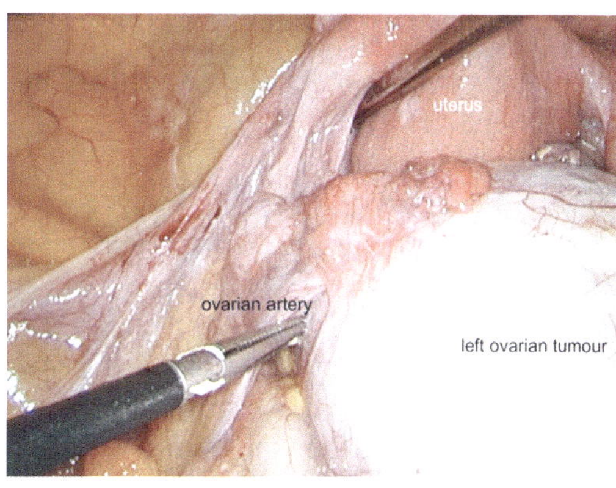

Fig. 5.1 Laparoscopic image showing uterus and left ovary

B. Díaz
Faculty of Medicine, Gynecology Oncology Unit, Institute Clinic of Gynecology, Obstetrics and Neonatology, Hospital Clinic de Barcelona, Institut d Investigacions Biomèdiques August Pi i Sunyer (IDIBAPS), University of Barcelona, Barcelona, Spain

Institut d'Investigacions Biomèdiques August Pi i Sunyer (IDIBAPS), Barcelona, Spain

B. Paño
Radiology Department, Hospital Clínic de Barcelona (CDI), Barcelona, Spain

P. Paredes
Institut d'Investigacions Biomèdiques August Pi i Sunyer (IDIBAPS), Barcelona, Spain

Faculty of Medicine, University of Barcelona, Barcelona, Spain

Nuclear Medicine Department, Hospital Clínic Barcelona (CDI), Barcelona, Spain

S. Vidal-Sicart (✉)
Institut d'Investigacions Biomèdiques August Pi i Sunyer (IDIBAPS), Barcelona, Spain

Nuclear Medicine, Hospital Clinic of Barcelona, Catalonia, Barcelona, Spain
e-mail: svidal@clinic.cat

A. Collarino et al. (eds.), *Nuclear Medicine Manual on Gynaecological Cancers and Other Female Malignancies*, https://doi.org/10.1007/978-3-031-05497-6_5

5.1.2 Routes of Spreading of Disease

Ovarian cancer is one of the most insidious cancers, due to its presentation and its pattern of spread (peritoneal, lymphatic, and hematogenous). The two first routes are the most important (responsible for about 90% of deaths in these patients). These routes are not mutually exclusive of each other.

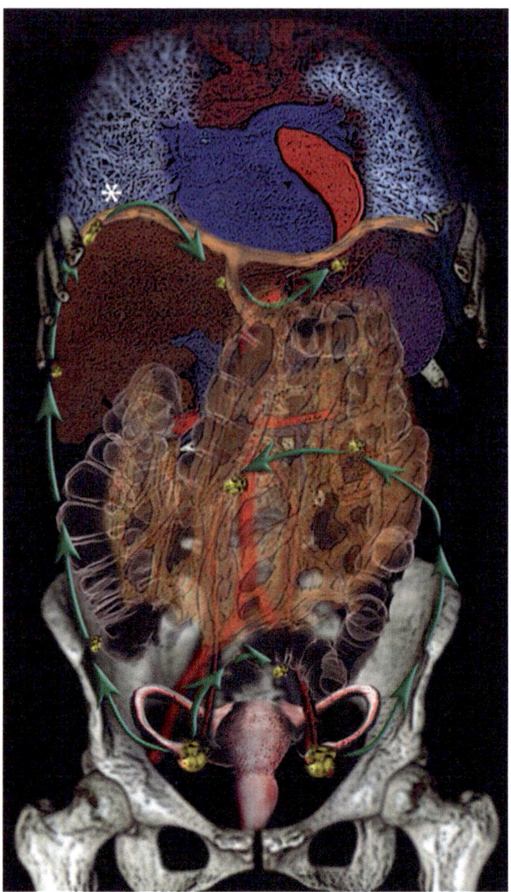

Fig. 5.2 Through respiratory movements, endoperitoneal fluid with neoplastic cells finally reaches all epithelial areas and especially the subphrenic space (right greater than left). (*) malignant cells in peritoneal fluid through the right hemidiaphragm, can embolize to lymphatic vessels resulting in pleural effusion

1. Peritoneal spread: The most common, premature, and characteristic route. Consists in invasion of the peritoneal blade towards the peritoneal cavity, where cancer cells will colonize the peritoneal surface with secondary invasion of the intraperitoneal organs.

   The exfoliated cells are distributed by gravity into the pouch of Douglas, and by the normal flow of peritoneal fluid throughout the peritoneal cavity, which is influenced by respiratory movements. The serous fluid circulates in the cavity and is preferentially drawn upward in the paracolic gutters to the right subphrenic space, where it is absorbed. The mesothelial cells of the right subphrenic peritoneum have wide intercellular gaps that facilitate absorption into the terminal lymphatics of the mediastinum.

   The common sites of peritoneal metastases in ovarian cancer:

   - Greater omentum
   - Right subphrenic space (diaphragm and liver Surface)
   - Paracolic gutters
   - Pouch of Douglas
   - Surface of the small and large bowel (Fig. 5.2)

2. The *para-aortic pathways* are one of the two main routes of spread of ovarian neoplasms.

   Lymph drains from the ovaries along two peduncles, one of which accompanies the ovarian blood vessels. Thus, the first retroperitoneal lymph nodes of this pathway are at the level of the renal hilum and differ depending on their laterality. Beyond these lymph nodes, metastatic cells spread in a retrograde direction toward the aortic bifurcation. This pathway bypasses the lymph nodes in the pelvis.

   The *lateral pelvic pathway* drains lymph from the pelvic organs to the external iliac lymph node group.

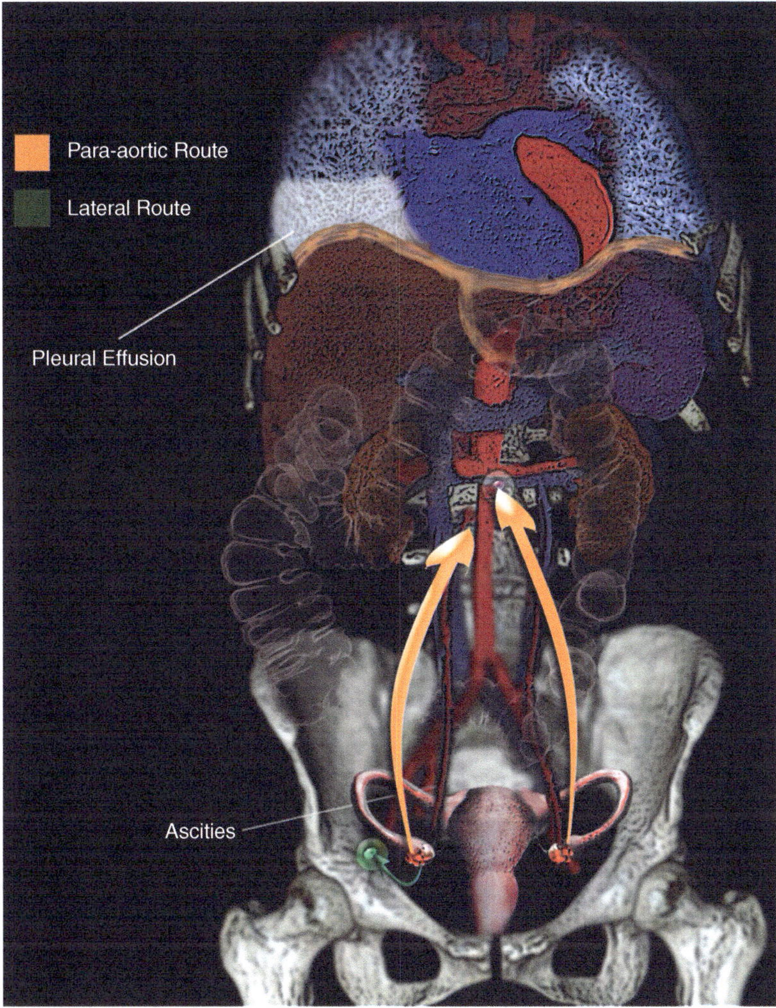

Fig. 5.3 Scheme representing the para-aortic and lateral pathways

The transdiaphragmatic communication of pleural and abdominal vessels causes pleural effusion and occlusion of lymphatic vessels causes ascites (Fig. 5.3).

3. Hematogenous spread: Occurs in advanced stages. In these cases, the most common is liver and lung infiltration (Fig. 5.4).

5.1.3 Tumor Types

Epithelial ovarian cancer is the sixth leading cause of death among women in Europe and the leading cause of death from gynecological cancer (approximately 65,000 new cases per year and 45,000 deaths). It is estimated that, worldwide in 15 years, the incidence of such neoplasia will increase by 55% and there will be an increase in mortality by 67%.

Ovarian cancer includes a wide variety of neoplasms that are histologically divided into three groups: epithelial, stromal, and germinal. Epithelial ovarian cancer (EOC) is the most common (90% of malignant ovarian tumors) and includes the following histological subtypes: high-grade serous, endometrioid, clear cells, low-grade serous, and mucinous.

The majority of patients with EOC (60–65%) are diagnosed in advanced stages or stage III/IV

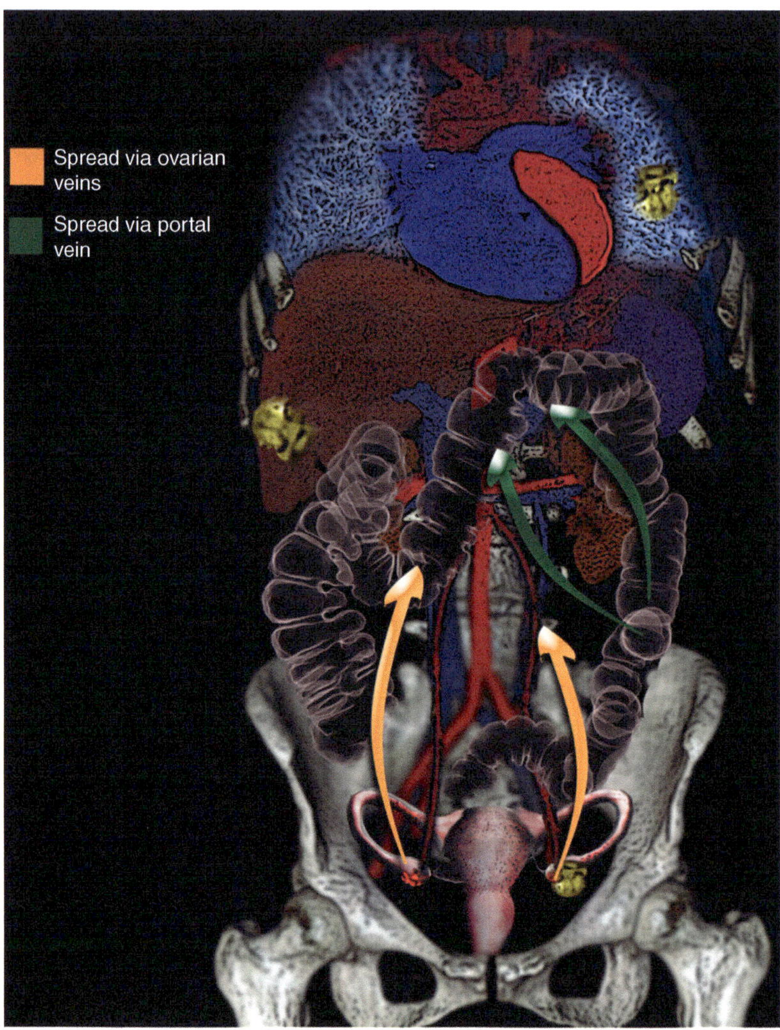

Fig. 5.4 Scheme of the main routes for hematogenous spread

of the FIGO (International Federation of Gynecology and Obstetrics) and undergo radical cytoreductive surgery and chemotherapy. Tumors diagnosed in the initial stage (stage I–II) require complete staging surgery to histologically assess the possible existence of peritoneal or lymph node disease.

Staging surgery in these cases includes bilateral anexectomy, hysterectomy, pelvic and paraaortic lymphadenectomy, omentectomy, and a complete examination with biopsies of the abdominal-pelvic cavity and the peritoneum. Systematic pelvic and paraaortic lymphadenectomy (from inguinal ligament to left renal vein) in stage I–II EOC is essential since confirming the presence of lymph node metastases means restaging the disease as stage III. This change of stage has important prognostic and therapeutic implications. Patients with initial clinical stage EOC have a lymph node involvement rate of 10–30% (average of 15%) [1–5].

5.1.4 FIGO and TNM Classification

There are two systems used for staging ovarian cancer: the FIGO (International Federation of Gynaecology and Obstetrics) system, which is the most commonly used, and the AJCC (American Joint Committee on Cancer) TNM staging system [6] (Table 5.1, Figs. 5.5 and 5.6).

Table 5.1 TNM and FIGO classifications (1)

Stage	TNM	FIGO stage	Stage description
I	T1 N0 M0	I	Tumor confined to ovaries or fallopian tube(s) (T1). It has not spread to nearby lymph nodes (N0) or to distant sites (M0).
IA	T1a N0 M0	IA	Tumor limited to one ovarian or fallopian tube (T1a). It has not spread to nearby lymph nodes (N0) or to distant sites (M0).
IB	T1b N0 M0	IB	Tumor limited to both ovarian (T1b). It has not spread to nearby lymph nodes (N0) or to distant sites (M0).
IC	T1C N0 M0	IC	Tumor limited to 1 or both ovaries or fallopian tubes, with any of the following: (T1c). It has not spread to nearby lymph nodes (N0) or to distant sites (M0)
	T1c1 N0 M0	IC1	Surgical spill (T1c1)
	T1c2 N0 M0	IC2	Capsule ruptured before surgery or tumor on ovarian or fallopian tube surface (T1c2)
	T1c3 N0 M0	IC3	Malignant cells in the ascites or peritoneal washings (T1c3).
II	T2 N0 M0	II	Tumor involves 1 or both ovaries or fallopian tubes with pelvic extension (below pelvic brim) or primary peritoneal cancer (T2) It has not spread to nearby lymph nodes (N0) or to distant sites (M0).
	T2a N0 M0	IIA	Extension and/or implants on uterus and/or fallopian tubes and/or ovaries (T2a).
	T2b N0 M0	IIB	Extension to other pelvic intraperitoneal tissues (T2b)
III	T1-2-3 N1 M0	III	Tumor involves 1 or both ovaries or fallopian tubes, or primary peritoneal cancer, with cytologically or histologically confirmed spread to the peritoneum outside the pelvis and/or metastasis to the retroperitoneal lymph nodes (T1/2-N1). It has not spread to n distant sites (M0).
IIIA	T3a1 N0/n1 M0	IIIA1	Positive retroperitoneal lymph nodes (only cytologically or histologically proven): IIIA1(i) metastasis up to 10 mm in greatest dimension IIIA1(ii) metastasis more than 10 mm in greatest dimension
	T1-T3a2 N0/N1 M0	IIIA2	IIIA2: Microscopic extrapelvic (above the pelvic brim) peritoneal involvement with or without positive retroperitoneal lymph nodes
IIIB	T3b N0/N1 M0	IIIB	Macroscopic peritoneal metastasis beyond the pelvis up to 2 cm in greatest dimension, with or without metastasis to the retroperitoneal lymph nodes.
IIIC	T3c N0/N M0		Macroscopic peritoneal metastasis beyond the pelvis more than 2 cm in greatest dimension, with or without metastasis to the retroperitoneal lymph nodes (includes extension of tumor to capsule of liver and spleen without parenchymal involvement of either organ).
IV	Any T Any N M1		Distant metastasis excluding peritoneal metastases.
	Any T Any N M1	IVA	Pleural effusion with positive cytology.
		IVB	Parenchymal metastases and metastases to extra-abdominal organs (including inguinal lymph nodes and lymph nodes outside of the abdominal cavity).

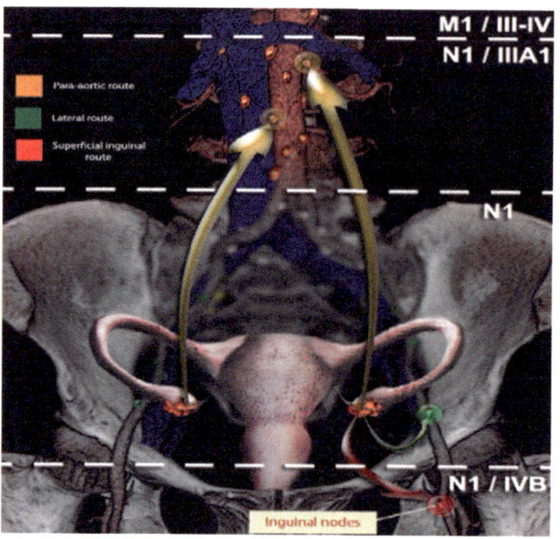

Fig. 5.5 Scheme of the main routes for lymphatic spread and their staging implication

- *Tracers*—Two different tracers have been used (Fig. 5.7):
  - Indocyanine green (ICG): 0.5 ml per injection site (Figs. 5.8 and 5.9).
  - Radiotracers ([^{99m}Tc]Tc-albumin nanocolloid): 0.2 ml, 37 MBq per injection site.
- Preliminary results (from systematic review):
  - Global detection rate: 97.6% (lumbo-aortic 83.3%, pelvic 43%).
  - Sensitivity: 66.7%.
  - Negative Predictive Value: 96.6%.
- On-going studies: there are two ongoing phase II clinical trials:
  - SENTOV study (using radiotracer and ICG)
  - SELLY study (based on ICG) [7–9] (Fig. 5.10)

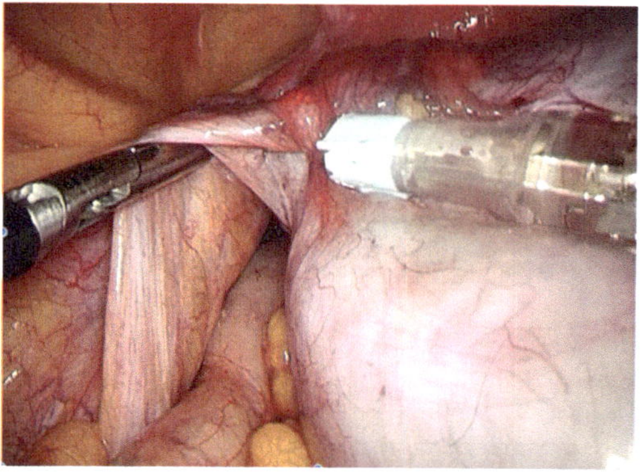

Fig. 5.6 Tracer injection in the infundibular ligament

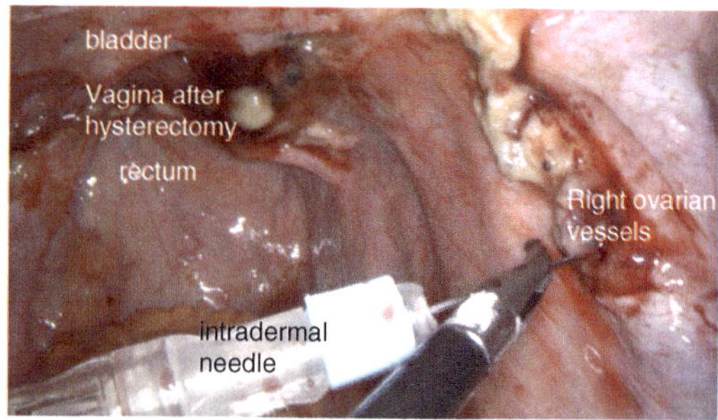

Fig. 5.7 Tracer injection in the right ovarian ligament stump

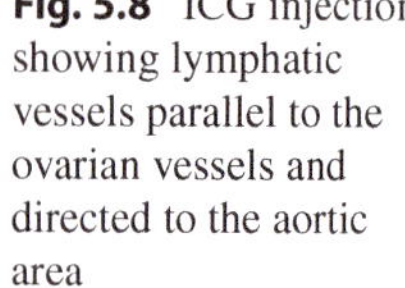

Fig. 5.8 ICG injection showing lymphatic vessels parallel to the ovarian vessels and directed to the aortic area

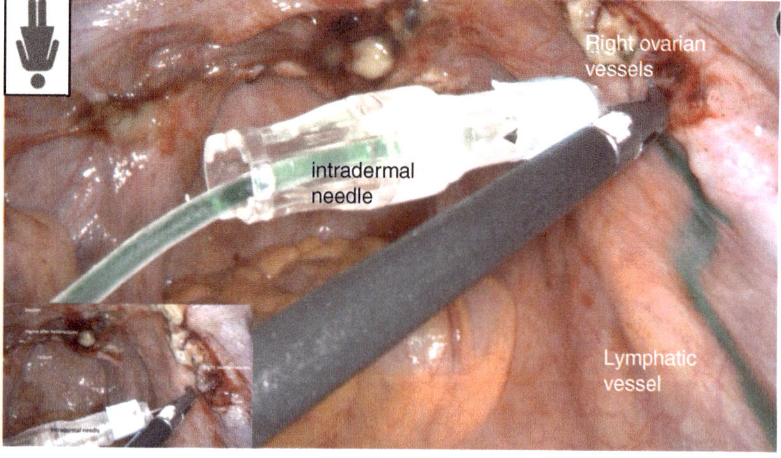

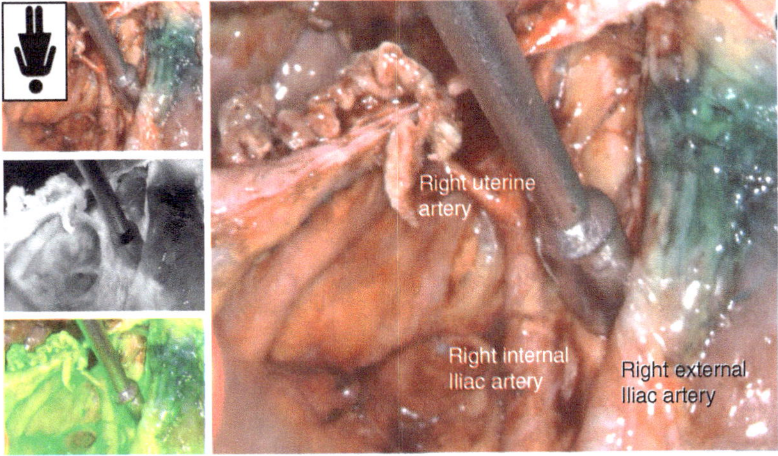

Fig. 5.9 Check-up right pelvic region using the gamma probe and the NIR camera

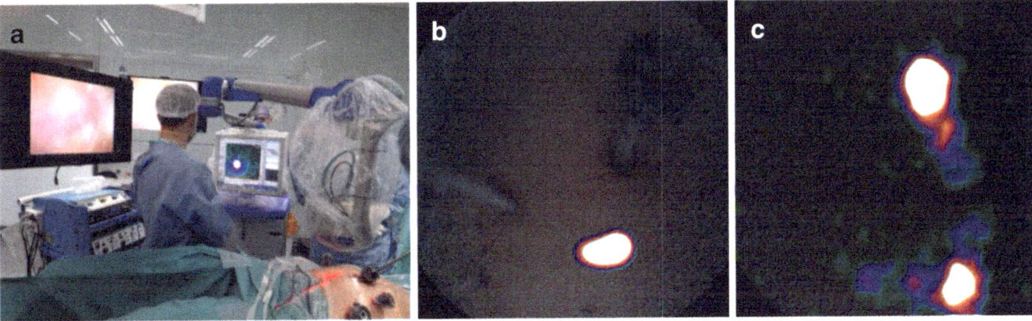

Fig. 5.10 (**a**) Portable gamma camera inside the OR (**b**–**c**) Images acquired with fused optical and scintigraphic image at 15 min p.i. (**b**, early study) and 60 min p.i. (**c**, late study)

5.2 Utility of CT, MR, and PET/CT

5.2.1 Role of Morphologic Imaging Techniques in Staging

US is the first diagnostic tool to detect an ovarian mass. If the mass is indeterminate at US, an MRI should be performed.

CT is the technique of choice for staging because of its wide availability and because a complete thoracoabdominal study can rapidly be acquired, with rates of diagnostic precision of 60%–90% for all stages. CT identifies eligible patients for complete cytoreductive surgery, establishes a precise mapping of peritoneal lesions, and anticipates possible surgical difficulties. CT has a low sensitivity (40%–43%) but a good specificity (89%–96%) for lymph node involvement. Furthermore, CT is the standard imaging technique for the evaluation of suspected recurrence (Fig. 5.11).

MR imaging using functional techniques is emerging as a technique that may be able to overcome limitations of staging CT. Sensitivity is higher for MRI (particularly using DW sequences) for implants smaller than 1 cm, in anatomic areas where small tumor implants are adjacent to tissues with similar signal intensity, in detecting small peritoneal implants, and in investigating bladder or rectal involvement. However, actually there is still a paucity of data on advanced MRI techniques for staging ovarian cancer.

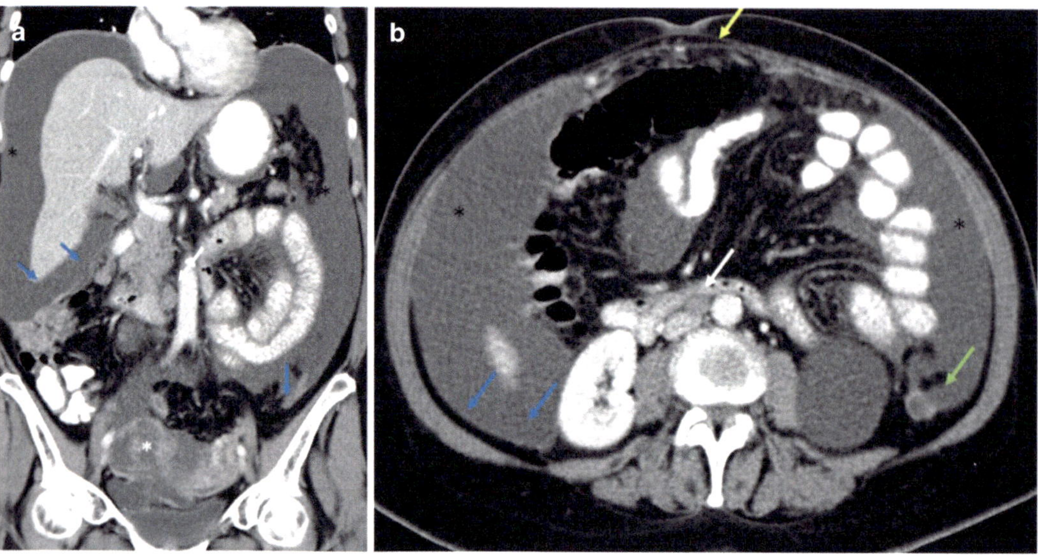

Fig. 5.11 Coronal (**a**) and axial (**b**) contrast-enhanced CT image in a 65-year-old woman with ovarian cancer shows right ovarian mass (7 cm) (White *). The patient shows signs of peritoneal tumor spread that include large amounts of ascites (black *), nodular stranding of the great omentum (yellow arrow), nodular implant (13 mm) (green arrow), and lineal thickening of the parietal omentum throughout the abdomen and pelvis (blue arrow). Note enlarged aortocaval lymph node of 11 mm (White arrow)

5.2.2 Role of Functional Imaging Techniques in Staging ([^{18}F]FDG PET/CT)

Surgical staging performing pelvic and para-aortic lymph node dissection is preferred for epithelial ovarian cancer. Sentinel lymph node biopsy could be an alternative but is not developed yet. Functional imaging techniques such as FDG PET/CT are not sensitive enough to replace surgical staging although the high negative predictive value, up to 96%, makes it an essential tool for diagnosis. Despite the low sensitivity for the detection of nodal involvement, the main contribution for staging is the detection of distant metastasis, extra-abdominal lesions, or lesions contraindicating primary cytoreduction, which provide a change in management and is associated with a worse prognosis. FDG PET/CT is especially useful in the detection of diaphragmatic lesions (Fig. 5.13) and reaches the highest agreement with surgical findings, of 78%. Instead, mesenteric nodules and miliary peritoneal disease are more frequently detected by CT.

Indications for FDG PET/CT in ovarian cancer:

- Suspicion of advanced disease: when IIIC /IV is suspected must be performed to discard distant metastases contraindicating primary cytoreduction.
- Non-conclusive lesions on other imaging techniques (CT or MRi) (Figs. 5.12, 5.13 and 5.14).

Methodology

- Contrast-enhanced CT for attenuation correction is preferred, but if not available PET with a low-dose CT is also indicated.
- Oral contrast helps in the evaluation of peritoneal serous bowel lesions.
- Coronal and sagittal reconstructions of abdominal sections are recommended [10–13].

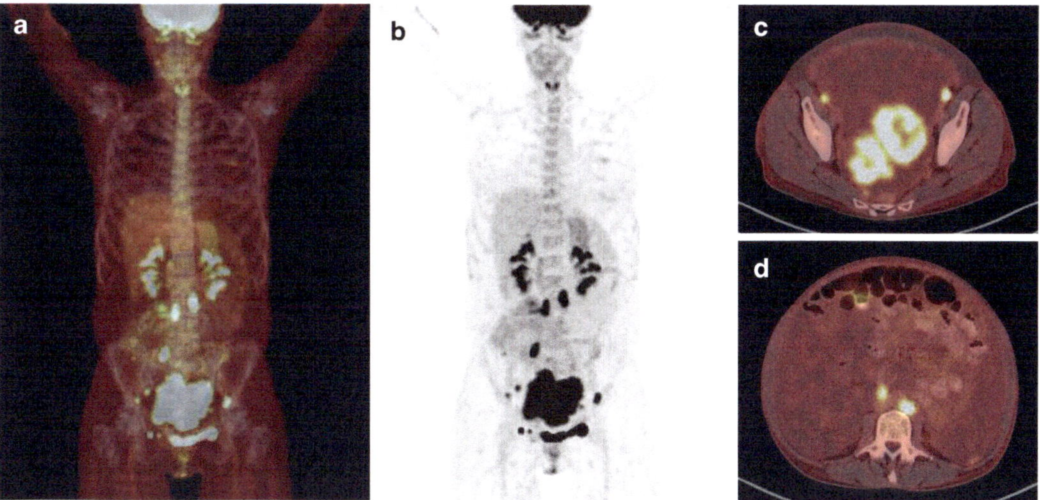

Fig. 5.12 FDG PET/CT performed for staging purposes on a 62-year-old woman with adnexial mass. Whole-body fused VTR/MPR (**a**) and MIP PET image (**b**) show pelvic hypermetabolic mass, with bilateral pelvic nodal (**c**), and para-aortic (**d**) nodal metastasis

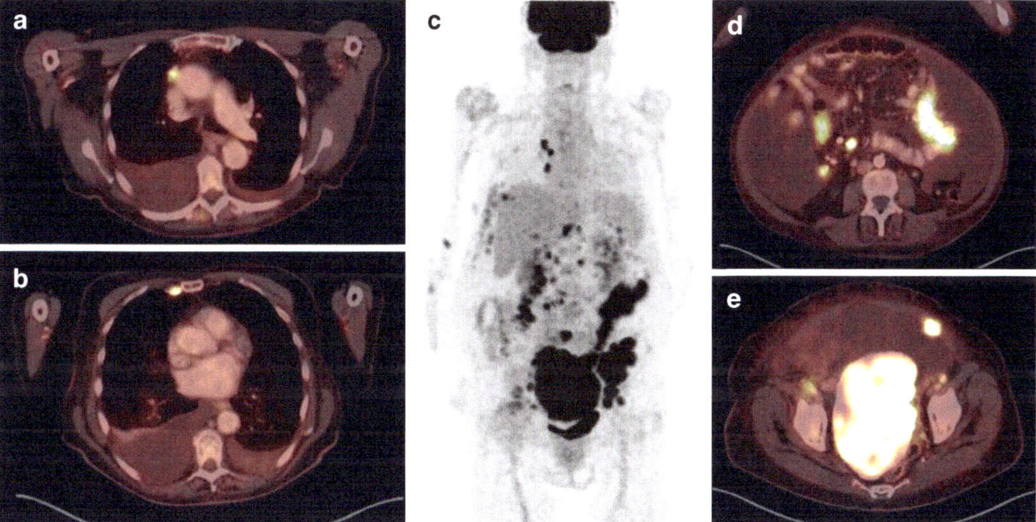

Fig. 5.13 FDG PET/CT performed for staging purposes. Whole-body MIP PET image (**c**) shows an adnexial mass suggesting ovarian cancer €, with peritoneal carcinomatosis (**d**) and extra-abdominal disease in a prevascular lymph node (**a**) and in the right internal mammary chain (**b**), ascites (**d**–**e**), and pleural effusion (**a**–**b**)

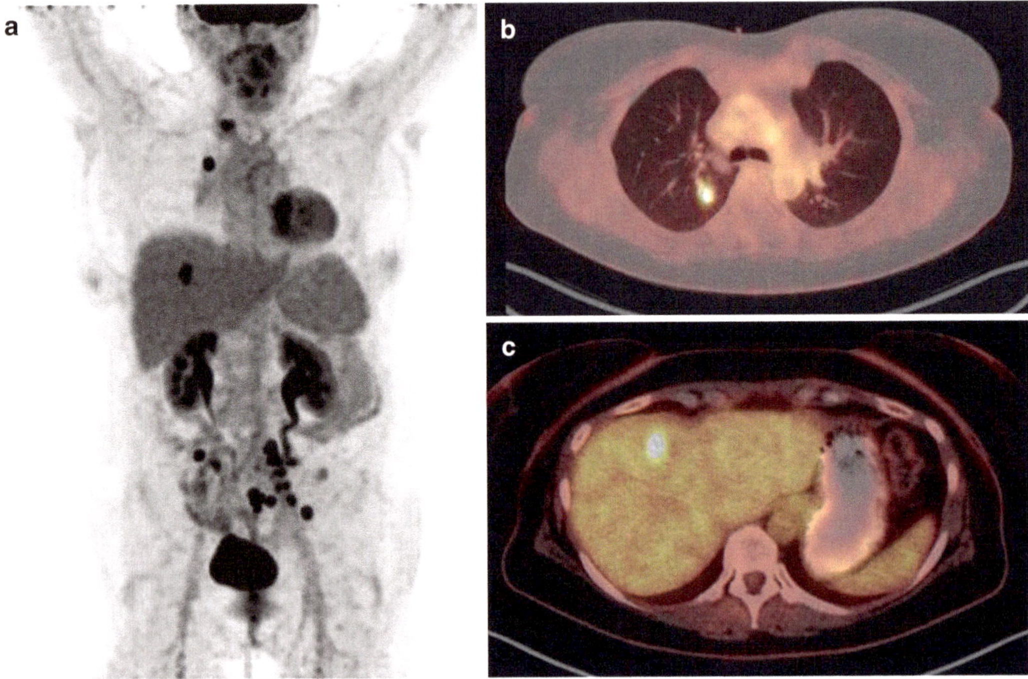

Fig. 5.14 FDG PET/CT performed for staging purposes. (**a**) MIP image. Distant metastases such as pulmonary nodules (**b**) or liver metastases (**c**) are less common but must be discarded

5.3 ROLL and/or RSL for Non-palpable Lesions Recurrences

Radioguided surgery technique has been successfully used in several clinical indications based on the accumulation of an injected radiotracer in a target lesion that is designed to be retained at the injection site (ROLL; Radioguided Occult Lesion Localization; RSL: Radioguided Seed Localization).

In the ROLL approach, part of the tracer used for sentinel lymph node biopsy is retained inside the lesion (if intratumorally injected) and it can be used to demarcate the primary lesion or its margins. However, the most widespread approach is the use of [99mTc]Tc-macroaggregate albumin (MAA), with high particle size, which avoids its lymphatic spread and can improve the local tracer retention.

Indications

Marking of non-palpable lesions (either benign or malignant).

Advantages

- The radiotracer can be injected into the lesion the day before or some hours prior to surgery.
- Localization of the lesion guided by a gamma detector probe (used in sentinel node).
- Reduction of dose of exposure to ionizing radiations among surgical personnel.
- Flexibility of surgical schedule.
- Shorter surgical time (one activity focus without radioactive background).

Disadvantages

– Tracer spreading depending on the particle size used (larger tissue resections).
– Non-accessible lesions to be injected (avoids technique).
– Non-nodular lesions (tracer diffusion).

Methodological Aspects for Injection (CT-Guided) and Resection (Probes, Other Devices…)

- Check the lesion in previous diagnostic images (CT, MRI, ultrasound, PET/CT).
- -Decide which imaging technique will be used for radiotracer injection (usually ultrasound or CT) and confirm the correct lesion localization.
- -Calculating the shortest distance between the skin and nodule while taking into account the tissues that will be passed through.
- An slow injection of 0.1–0.2 mL of [99mTc] Tc-MAA (37–74 MBq, depending on the day of injection) is given.
- 0.2 mL of radiopaque contrast medium or 0.1–0.3 mL of air (for needle lavage) can be given.
- Verification of the administration may be carried out in two ways:
  – An image verifies that the contrast medium (if used) is in place.
  – The most used approach is performing a scintigraphic image (ideally with SPECT/CT) to rule out the potential tracer spillage.
- A skin mark could be helpful in some lesions (especially superficial).
- During surgery (open or laparoscopic) the gamma probe must be strategically placed and an accurate scanning of the zone should be performed to identify the focus of greatest radioactivity.
- After removal of lesion, absence of residual activity in the surgical field should be confirmed (Fig. 5.15) [14–17].

5.4 Radioguided Seed Localization

This procedure uses a sealed titanium capsule (4x0.8 mm) that fits within a 18-G needle containing a nontherapeutic low dose of 125I (usually 7 MBq). RSL has mostly been applied in breast cancer patients for tumor resection (like ROLL) and, especially in those receiving neoadjuvant treatment.

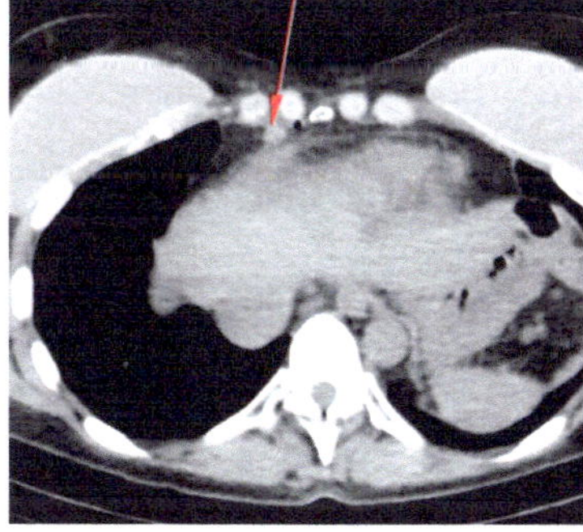
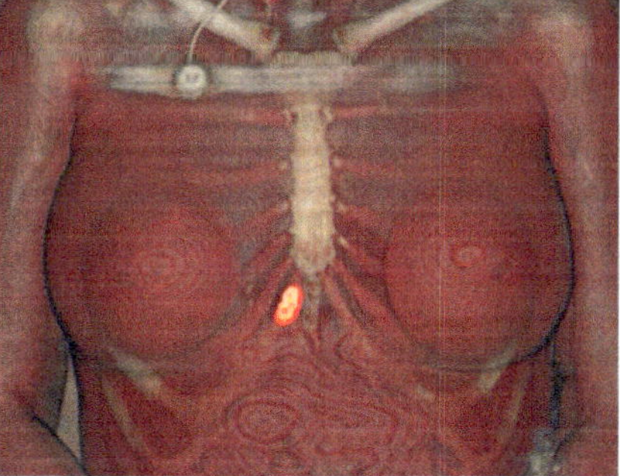
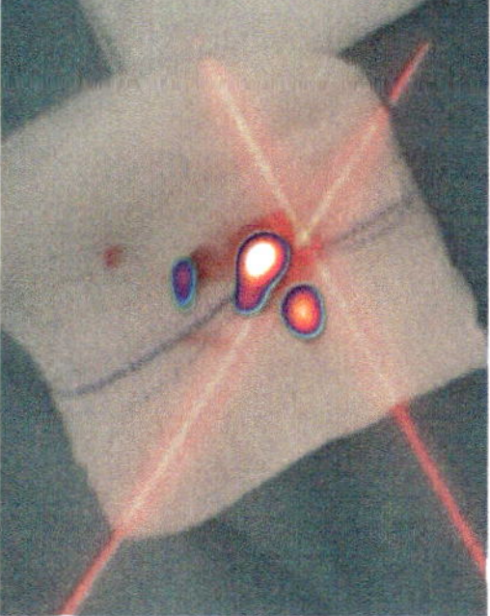

Fig. 5.15 ROLL technique. Patient with an enlarged cardiophrenic lymph node (in CT image on the left) with a significant uptake in PET/CT scan. After injection of 37 MBq in 0.2 ml of [99mTc]Tc-Albumin macroaggregates a SPECT/CT was performed (central view showing volume rendering image with the activity in the lymph node). The node was retrieved with laparoscopic approach. Left-hand side image shows the excised node activity assessed with a portable gamma camera

Advantages

- Sealed radioactive source (no spillage).
- Flexibility in surgery timing (from several to same-day prior to surgery).
- Low radiation.
- Improved definition of the incision site.
- High reliability of intraoperatively target detection.

Disadvantages

- Regulatory issues.
- Potential loss of the seed.
- Not always possible to be introduced into the lesion.

Methodological aspects for injection (CT-guided) and resection (probes, other devices…).

- Check the lesion in previous diagnostic images (CT, MRI, ultrasound, PET/CT).
- Decide which imaging technique will be used for injection (ultrasound or CT) and confirm the correct lesion localization.
- Calculating the shortest distance between the skin and nodule while taking into account the tissues that will be passed through.
- A 18-gauge needle, long enough for the injection is used. The tip of the needle is covered by bone wax (to avoid seed's fall).
- Continuous monitoring with ultrasound probe (or CT control) is performed.
- When needle's tip position is adequate the guide of the needle is pushed in order to release the seed.
- Verification of the administration may be carried out by on-site ultrasound or radiologic image. Moreover, a scintigraphic image with a gamma camera is usually done (set up in a 27-KeV energy photopeak). With these images, the adequate seed position in the lesion is assessed (especially in SPECT/CT fused images).
- A skin mark could be helpful in some lesions (especially superficial).
- During surgery (open or laparoscopic) the gamma probe (with isotope selection set at 125I energy) plays an accurate scanning of the zone should be performed to identify the focus of radioactivity.
- Once localized, the surgeon dissects the tissues and nuclear medicine staff verifies with the probe that the radioactive focus is properly addressed.
- Absence of residual activity in the surgical field should be confirmed [18–22] (Figs. 5.16, 5.17, 5.18, 5.19, 5.20 and 5.21).

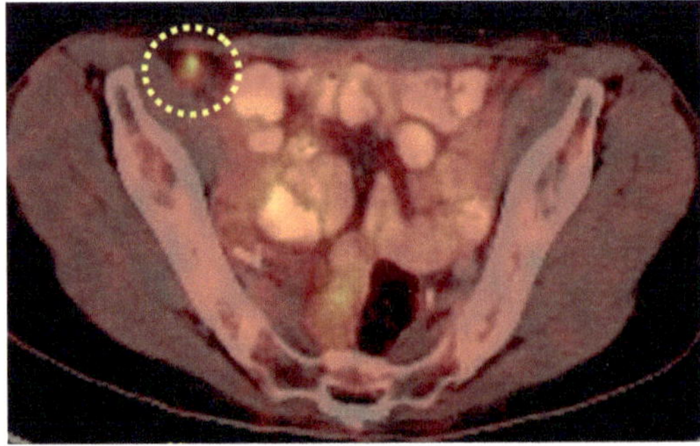

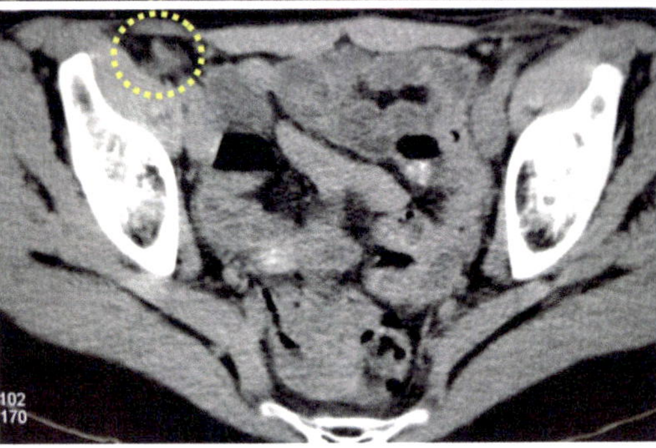

Fig. 5.16 PET/CT fused images (up) and CT images (down), belonging to a patient with an implant from ovarian origin in her pelvic right side (dotted circles)

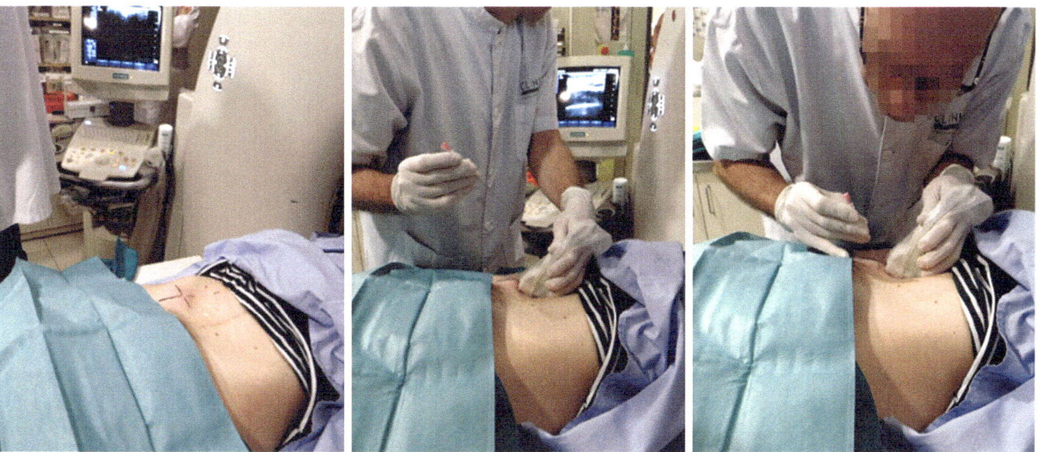

Fig. 5.17 RSL/ROLL approach. Ultrasound-guided injection in a patient with an ovarian implant below muscle rectus abdominis. Both markers can be positioned within the lesion with this technique

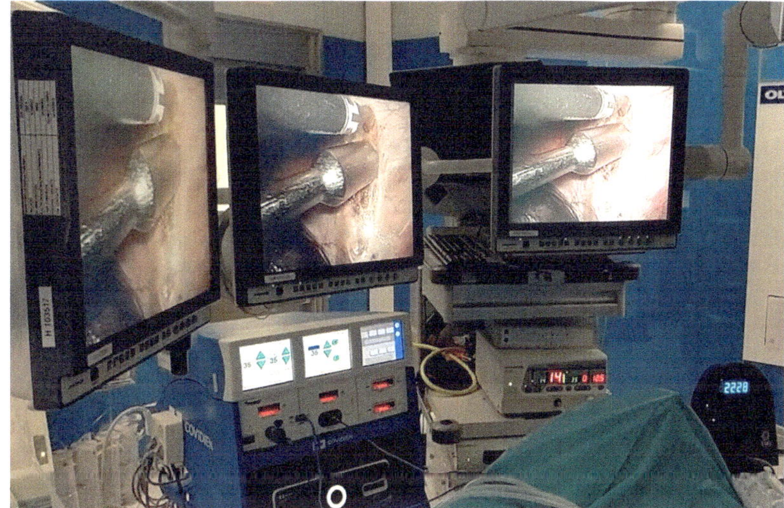

Fig. 5.18 Laparoscopic approach in a RSL surgery. The gamma probe (laparoscopic) points to the area with high activity (visualized in the device at the bottom of right-hand side), corresponding, in this case, to an iodine seed

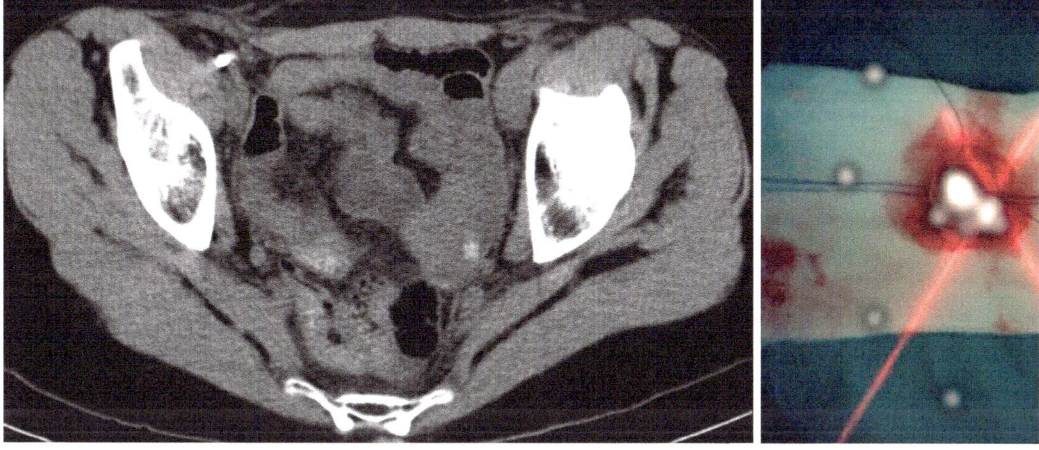

Fig. 5.19 The 125I seed is visualized on the right-hand side in the CT scan (left). After excision, its activity is depicted (using the 125I photopeak energy) with a portable gamma camera (right)

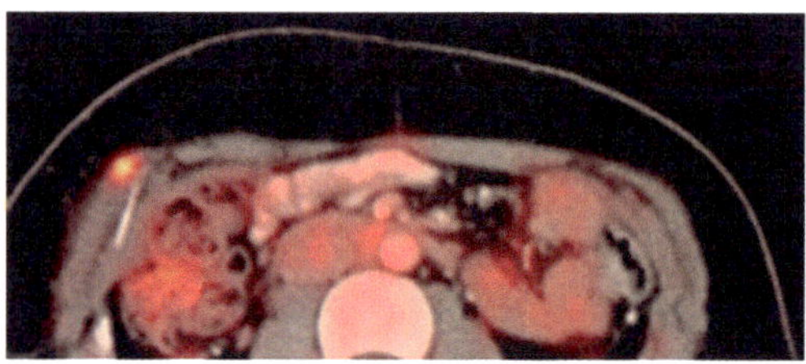

Fig. 5.20 Right Oblique muscle implant from ovarian cancer. Preoperative [18F]18F-FDG PET/CT scan (fused and native images are provided), showed a well-defined uptake within the muscle body. Biopsy found a metastatic deposit of ovarian origin

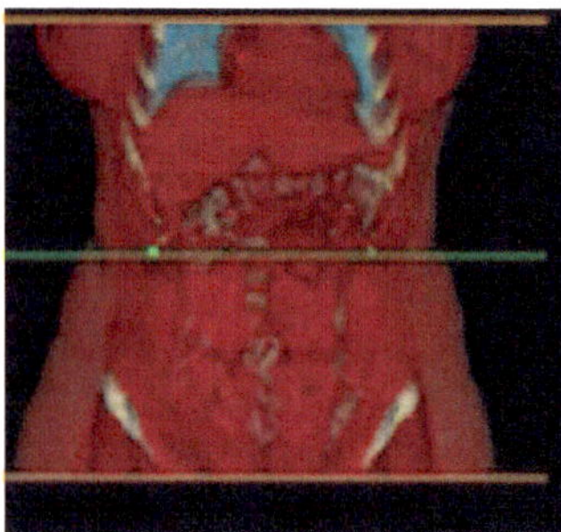

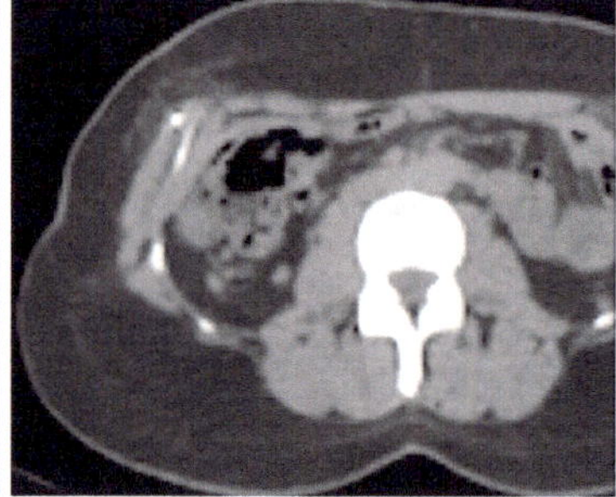

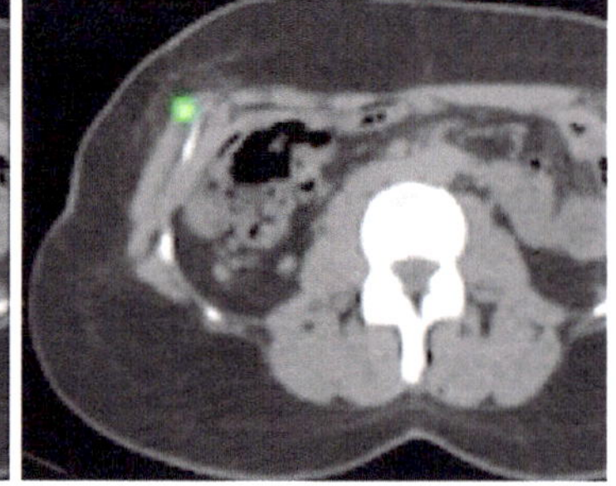

Fig. 5.21 RSL approach. After ultrasound guidance, a 125I seed was introduced into the lesion. SPECT/CT with volumetric rendering (left) and fused images (right) showed that 125I seed was correctly placed into the lesion

References

1. Colombo N, Sessa C, du Bois A, Ledermann J, McCluggage WG, McNeish I, Morice P, Pignata S, Ray-Coquard I, Vergote I, Baert T, Belaroussi I, Dashora A, Olbrecht S, Planchamp F, Querleu D. ESMO-ESGO ovarian cancer consensus conference working group. ESMO-ESGO consensus conference recommendations on ovarian cancer: pathology and molecular biology, early and advanced stages, borderline tumours and recurrent disease†. Ann Oncol. 2019;30:672–705. https://doi.org/10.1093/annonc/mdz062.
2. Paño B, Sebastià C, Ripoll E, Paredes P, Salvador R, Buñesch L, Nicolau C. Pathways of lymphatic spread in gynecologic malignancies. Radiographics. 2015;35:916–45. https://doi.org/10.1148/rg.2015140086.
3. Park HJ, Kim DW, Yim GW, Nam EJ, Kim S, Kim YT. Staging laparoscopy for the management of early-stage ovarian cancer: a metaanalysis. Am J Obstet Gynecol. 2013;209(58):e1–8. https://doi.org/10.1016/j.ajog.2013.04.013.
4. Torre LA, Trabert B, DeSantis CE, Miller KD, Samimi G, Runowicz CD, Gaudet MM, Jemal A, Siegel RL. Ovarian cancer statistics, 2018. CA Cancer J Clin. 2018;68:284–96. https://doi.org/10.3322/caac.21456.
5. World Health Organization. The Global Cancer Observatory: Globocan; 2018. http://gco.iarc.fr/
6. Prat J, FIGO Committee on Gynecologic Oncology Obstet Gynecol Staging Classification for Cancer of the Ovary, Fallopian Tube, and Peritoneum: Abridged Republication of Guidelines From the International Federation of Gynecology and Obstetrics (FIGO). 2015;126:171–4. https://doi.org/10.1097/AOG.0000000000000917.
7. Lago V, Bello P, Matute L, Padilla-Iserte P, Marina T, Agudelo M, Domingo S. Sentinel lymph node technique in apparent early ovarian cancer: laparoscopic technique. J Minim Invasive Gynecol. 2020;27:1019–20. https://doi.org/10.1016/j.jmig.2019.09.790.
8. Scambia G, Nero C, Uccella S, Vizza E, Ghezzi F, Cosentino F, Chiantera V, Fagotti A. Sentinel-node biopsy in early stage ovarian cancer: a prospective multicentre study (SELLY). Int J Gynecol Cancer. 2019;29:1437–9. https://doi.org/10.1136/ijgc-2019-000886.
9. Uccella S, Zorzato PC, Lanzo G, Fagotti A, Cianci S, Gallina D, Gueli Alletti S, Monterossi G, Franchi M, Ghezzi F, Zannoni GF, Scambia G. The role of sentinel node in early ovarian cancer: a systematic review. Minerva Med. 2019;110:358–66. https://doi.org/10.23736/S0026-4806.19.06145-7.
10. Fruscio R, Sina F, Dolci C, Signorelli M, Crivellaro C, Dell'Anna T, Cuzzocrea M, Guerra L, Milani R, Messa C. Preoperative 18F-FDG PET/CT in the

management of advanced epithelial ovarian cancer. Gynecol Oncol. 2013;131:689–93. https://doi.org/10.1016/j.ygyno.2013.09.024.
11. Hynninen J, Kemppainen J, Lavonius M, Virtanen J, Matomäki J, Oksa S, Carpén O, Grénman S, Seppänen M, Auranen A. A prospective comparison of integrated FDG-PET/contrast-enhanced CT and contrast-enhanced CT for pretreatment imaging of advanced epithelial ovarian cancer. Gynecol Oncol. 2013;131:389–94. https://doi.org/10.1016/j.ygyno.2013.08.023.
12. Lee IO, Lee JY, Kim HJ, Nam EJ, Kim S, Kim SW, Lee CY, Kang WJ, Kim YT. Prognostic significance of supradiaphragmatic lymph node metastasis detected by ^{18}F-FDG PET/CT in advanced epithelial ovarian cancer. BMC Cancer. 2018;18:1165. https://doi.org/10.1186/s12885-018-5067-1.
13. Schmidt S, Meuli RA, Achtari C, Prior JO. Peritoneal carcinomatosis in primary ovarian cancer staging: comparison between MDCT, MRI, and 18F-FDGPET/CT. Clin Nucl Med. 2015;40:371–7. https://doi.org/10.1097/RLU.0000000000000768.
14. Bowles H, Sánchez N, Tapias A, Paredes P, Campos F, Bluemel C, Valdés Olmos RA, Vidal-Sicart S. Radioguided surgery and the GOSTT concept: from pre- operative image and intraoperative navigation to image-assisted excision. Rev Esp Med Nucl Imagen Mol. 2017;36:175–84. https://doi.org/10.1016/j.remn.2016.09.004.
15. Chan BK, Wiseberg-Firtell JA, Jois RH, Jensen K, Audisio RA. Localization techniques for guided surgical excision of non-palpable breast lesions. Cochrane Database Syst Rev. 2015;31:CD009206. https://doi.org/10.1002/14651858.CD009206.
16. Manca G, Garau LM, Romanini A, Rubello D, Nuzzo A, Barbarello L, Fantechi L, Colletti PM, Boggi U, Volterrani D. Detection of uterine Leiomyosarcoma peritoneal lesions by SPECT/CT and ROLL technique. Clin Nucl Med. 2019;44:826–8. https://doi.org/10.1097/RLU.0000000000002725.
17. Manca G, Mazzarri S, Rubello D, Tardelli E, Delgado-Bolton RC, Giammarile F, Roncella M, Volterrani D, Colletti PM. Radioguided occult lesion localization: technical procedures and clinical applications. Clin Nucl Med. 2017;42:e498–503. https://doi.org/10.1097/RLU.0000000000001858.
18. Bortz MD, Khokar A, Winchester DJ, Moo-Young TA, Ecanow DB, Ecanow JS, Prinz RA. Radioactive iodine-125 seed localization as an aid in reoperative neck surgery. Am J Surg. 2021;221:534–7. https://doi.org/10.1016/j.amjsurg.2020.12.048.
19. Garner HW, Bestic JM, Peterson JJ, Attia S, Wessell DE. Preoperative radioactive seed localization of nonpalpable soft tissue masses: an established localization technique with a new application. Skelet Radiol. 2017;46:209–16. https://doi.org/10.1007/s00256-016-2529-x.
20. Hassing CMS, Tvedskov TF, Kroman N, Klausen TL, Drejøe JB, Tvedskov JF, Lambine TL, Kledal H, Lelkaitis G, Langhans L. Radioactive seed localisation of non-palpable lymph nodes - a feasibility study. Eur J Surg Oncol. 2018;44:725–30. https://doi.org/10.1016/j.ejso.2018.02.211.
21. Jakub J, Gray R. Starting a radioactive seed localization program. Ann Surg Oncol. 2015;22:3197–202. https://doi.org/10.1245/s10434-015-4719-5.
22. Valdés Olmos RA, Vidal-Sicart S, Manca G, Mariani G, León-Ramírez LF, Rubello D, Giammarile F. Advances in radioguided surgery in oncology. Q J Nucl Med Mol Imaging. 2017;61:247–70. https://doi.org/10.23736/S1824-4785.17.02995-8.

GPSR Compliance

The European Union's (EU) General Product Safety Regulation (GPSR) is a set of rules that requires consumer products to be safe and our obligations to ensure this.

If you have any concerns about our products, you can contact us on ProductSafety@springernature.com

In case Publisher is established outside the EU, the EU authorized representative is:

Springer Nature Customer Service Center GmbH
Europaplatz 3
69115 Heidelberg, Germany

Batch number: 10371063

Printed by Printforce, the Netherlands